Breast **Cancer**

Behind the Scenes

Dana Conway

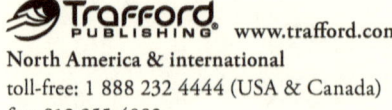 www.trafford.com
North America & international
toll-free: 1 888 232 4444 (USA & Canada)
fax: 812 355 4082

Contents

Acknowledgments

OF course here is where you talk about all of your inspiration and so forth and thank all of the people that sometimes to me, just doesn't make any sense whatsoever because there are people that you have no idea who or what they have to do with anything. So, in light of that, here it goes.

Foremost:
    I'd have to say Thank God!
Thank you to my family. I have named several in the book, but their names deserve special mention:
    My Son: Caleb Perez
    My Mom: Betty Conway
    My Dad: Isaac Conway

    My Brother: David Conway
    His Wife: Kristie Conway
        Their Children:
            David Conway II
            Dallas Conway
            Christopher Conway

There have been some additions to our family that have been blessings along the way.

Ashley Conway, and our precious Celestra born 12-14-10
Dhyana Coil who gave us our joyous little Avani born 12-22-12

My wonderful cousin, Denise McConnell. Thank you so, so much for giving up your time with your family to come up here and take care of me. I couldn't have asked for better care. I love my whole family, extended each and every one.

I couldn't have made it through without my best friend Cheryl Krug-Laskey. Everyone should be as lucky to have such a friend, we have been friends for 30 years now as well as the following two that I will mention, but Cheryl and I have a long history of, shall we say "information" that shall go to the grave about each other. That is scary, yet what a friend. Along those lines, I hold friendships dear, so I mustn't leave out Patti Mort, Kathy Boyd,(my other two friends of 30 years) and Thresea Smith.

I have so many more, but I better stop while I can. I love all of my friends, and don't know what I'd do without any of you!.

Now for some of the important people who helped save my life! My physicians:

Dr. Joyce Schofield – My Internal Medicine Physician, who had the joy of telling me I had cancer. This woman is remarkable. I can trust that she will be more than thorough with anything and everything that could come up with me. She has the kindest heart, and a warm personality. I truly have great respect for her knowledge, her compassion, and her willingness to go that extra mile. The Staff couldn't be more helpful and courteous.

Dr. Brad Storm – My Plastic Surgeon. What a kind, gentle, caring, man. His goal was, and still continues to be what is best for me, yet it's MY decision, and he supports that decision no matter what. I have always been treated with respect and care, no matter how big or small of an issue. He is here just to help me. His staff has such upbeat and helpful, and polite attitudes, you just feel right at home.

Dr. Prasanth Reddy – My Oncologist. I cannot say enough kind things about this man. Just think of all of the patients he can't save? What a burden for a person to bear. I truly believe he puts his whole heart and soul into finding a way to save everyone. He always greets his patient with a hug. His attention to detail is remarkable, and his knowledge far exceeds anything I could possibly "google." His staff, especially Krista, are always on their toes, making calls, and showing that you are cared for. I saw many people come and go, and still do, that don't always receive the best of news, and they don't always react with a smile on their face exactly. We have to literally put our lives in their hands and trust them. So, imagine your job, every day, facing people who quite possibly are going to die? Now, try being as pleasant as you can to each of them knowing that this is a possibility, and trying not to get personally attached or let it affect your job. I think it would be extraordinarily difficult, and I say CHEERS to you all!

Dr. Elizabeth Long – General Surgeon. Well, Dr. Long and I have had the pleasure of doing business several times before this occasion, and a few after. She is one of the few people that I know that ALWAYS has a smile on her face. It's like it's painted on there, then you can't help be happy and smile back. When I was diagnosed with breast cancer, we had a meeting. My parents, my son, myself and of course Dr. Long, who gently took us through the process of how things would "go down" from here. It cannot be an easy job for her either. I'm certain she faces many life and death situations all the time. That smile, it's always there, to comfort you. She has an amazing staff as well. They are all on top of every situation. As a patient, and being in an Office Manager Position myself, I can be a little judgmental of how different offices do things. I am not disappointed with ANY of my doctors. This must mean that they chose their staff well. As a patient, I can only say that I appreciate all the hard work that everyone does.

Now that I have my Physicians all covered, my family, and, my really close friends, I have two more people to thank.

Brian Joyce. Brian I almost can't find the words, you found them for me when I just couldn't. You listened to me when I whined about my stomach hurting, or any other aches and pains. Not to mention all the emotional business I was going through. I cannot begin to tell you how much I appreciate all the support that you have given me all these years. Your thoughtfulness will never be forgotten. Much love goes to you for all you've done for me.

You'll see in the book that Rebecca Sharp took the final photos. This is one of those things that just fell into place. I had never met Rebecca before, but I saw some of her work. She does very tasteful work. I got her information and we spoke. I asked if she would take the photos for me, and she was delighted to do so. As mentioned in the book, one of the hardest things for her to do, was to "not glamorize" me, or Photoshop things. I want the real thing. I wanted to make certain that what you are seeing in the book represents without a doubt, what the final result is after a mastectomy. I think she did an awesome job. If you need someone to glamorize you, she's your gal!

Rebecca Sharp
Sharp Images
http://www.rebeccasharpimages.com/
http://www.imageofawoman.com/
816-516-2822

Thanks Bec! You Rock!

FINALLY, I want to thank Eva and Don Acher. Without their help, my dream of getting this book published would never have happened. I don't believe that my connection with Eva and Don was by accident. I met them both on their wedding day in April 2013. I was their photographer, site unseen. Eva was a member of my parent's church. Eva and Don met at the Retirement Villa they were both staying at. Eva, who had been widowed for many years, and Don who had lost his wife not too many years prior, are complete opposites in many ways. But, you can't choose who you fall in love with, even at the age of 83 I suppose! So, on this day in April, when Miss Eva walked into the room where I would photograph her, I immediately loved her. I felt as if I'd known her my whole life. After the wedding and the settlement with the photo's we still continued to talk, and became even closer. Seems that our lives paralleled in many ways. However, what intrigued me the most about her was that she was a Holocaust Survivor. As one conversation led to another, she informed me that she had a book that was written in France, and she had it translated to an English version, but it was only released to some school libraries, and her wish was to get it published. I told her that I could help her with that. She was thrilled. So, as much as I'm excited about my book, I'm even MORE excited about Eva's book. So, please look for her book as well, Eva Rappart-Edmands-Acher Title "Hiding Through The Holocaust" Sub title "from buttercup fields to killing fields." I promise it is a story you will want to know about, and appreciate. So, THANK YOU EVA AND DON ACHER for being my friends, my adopted parents, my supporters, and making this possible! Cheers to you! Love you!

Preface

I decided to write this book when I was knee-deep in cancer mode. If you have breast cancer, then you know what I mean. I was determined to do this to help others.

One thing I will make clear from the start is there are no two people going through this situation that will have the same exact results. It just isn't possible. So this book is about *me*. I know; how conceited. Well, I am the least conceited person I know, but I really want to give some reference for *you*. I want to give you some *hope* that things can be OK. I want you to have *faith* that you can make it through this. I want you to know that there is someone out there that *loves* you. Trust me, someone does. I don't even know you, and I do.

These are my favorite words, and I gather strength from them every day: *hope, faith,* and *love*. First, you must always have *hope*. Hope is what carries us on; hope is what gives us those butterflies in our stomachs! Hope is the future! Second, if we have *faith* in our doctors, in ourselves to fight, in our families, in God, or whatever entity you believe in, then *faith* can give us the strength to look that crazy cancer in the eye and say *"Ha!"* Finally, *love*—love for others and for ourselves. *"Let your love shine!"* Even though you might have cancer, that doesn't mean you can't show love or receive it.

Now I'll tell you a little bit about my cancer story. I know; you hear everyone's once you tell somebody you have it. However, I want you to know my specifics. It was *so* important to me to find out all the information that I could when I was diagnosed. This is the basis of my book. When I found out that I had breast cancer, I did what almost everyone these days does: I searched the Internet for answers. *Wow!* A *lot* of information, yet *not*. I wanted to know most specifically this: *what am I going to look like?*

I could find before and after pictures. I could find pictures of women who had total mastectomies and no reconstruction. I could find little to no information about what happens when you have chemotherapy.

I mean, *what happens?* I could find enormous amounts of journal entries from doctors and a mind-boggling amount of big words that I didn't know the meanings of.

I love my plastic surgeon! He had a video for me and my family to watch, but still I had unanswered questions—questions that he could only answer with "Well, everyone's situation is different," which is true—very true!

So my quest is this. I took pictures from the very beginning, the day prior to my surgery, and periodically through my recovery until now, three years later. I wanted to show the progression of the healing. I want you to know what I felt like, what it was like during the healing, what it was like during the chemo—all the things that I could think of that I had questions about.

I hope that you find it helpful.

Please continue with caution! These pictures are *graphic*!

If they are too much for you, I'm sorry. I did group those pictures into one chapter, so you can just skip it if you don't want to see.

Again, I am trying to *help* you in your cancer journey. I think if you *want* to read *everything*, *great*. If you just want to look up a certain section in your research, *great*. It really is about what you need answers to.

I am proud to say that I am still cancer-free and the odds are good for me. I hope that you can fight with all your might and that your results are the best they can be.

Remember *hope*, *faith*, and *love*. Just know that cancer can change you, but it doesn't have to *define* you. You are you. Cancer is just a piece of your life now—a clip out of a scene in a movie, if you will. The reel will keep rolling, and so will you!

Good luck to you in whatever you are facing.

I will make every effort to write as much as I can. However, if you are like me, you want answers to certain questions and want them *now*. So as you see, I've broken this book down into a few simple sections for you. If you read the book from beginning to end, you will find some repetition as, like I said, I want you to be able to go to one section and get the answer you are looking for without having to read the whole book if you don't want to. So please forgive me for repeating myself. (*No*, I didn't have a memory lapse, and yes, I *do* have chemo brain!)

1. The biopsy (Well, unforgettable!)
2. My cancer details (This will give you the specifics about my kind of cancer, my treatment options, etc.)
3. Surgery (What you can expect.)

4. Pictures of my progression (I had a total mastectomy of my left breast with a TRAM reconstruction and reconstruction of the right breast.)

5. Chemo information (*Wow.* If you are facing chemo, it is extremely frightening. I will tell you all about the wonderful world of chemo!)

6. My cancer story (Some of you might want to know all the gory details of my life and how I found my cancer and all the other things that were going on at the same time. If you want to know more about my story, feel free to read this.)

7. *Caregivers* (What they go through!)

Chapter 1

"The Biopsy"

I guarantee you that there are dates that you never forget, and the day that you are diagnosed with cancer is one of those. I was officially diagnosed on my daddy's birthday, October 7, 2010.

I found a lump in my left breast on September 28, 2010. It was in a very odd place and felt very different than, say, a cyst or fibrocystic tumor.

I *just* had a mammogram in July with an *"All clear,"* so finding the lump was just a fluke thing. I was outside, and it was a little chilly, so I had my arms crossed to keep myself warm; that was when I felt the lump very close to the nipple area. First, I thought, *Nah, it's nothing. I just had a mammogram.* All still while I was outside, I was sort of fondling my breast in a sneaky sort of way so that the neighbors wouldn't notice! But no, this just didn't feel right.

I was living at home with my parents at the time. (I'm a forty-nine-year-old woman, was forty-five then, and yes, I am living with my parents!) I stepped inside and, oddly enough, asked my mother to feel the lump.

We lost my aunt to breast cancer years ago (my mother's oldest sister, Aunt Ruby), and she *made* us feel her lump. I know; weird, huh?

Actually, it probably saved my life. Knowing the difference between a cyst and a cancer lump is extremely helpful.

Having this knowledge, my mother looked at me with this semiworried look and said, "Hmmm, that really doesn't feel right, does it?" I told her no. We both decided we'd wait until the next day before we got too riled up about it.

Well, the next day came, and the lump was still there. So it was decided that I would call my doctor on Monday.

Monday came, and the call was made. There was little time wasted. I got in to see her rather quickly and got a mammogram and a sonogram of the breast within a day or so. The radiologist was concerned. They wanted me to see my doctor and have a biopsy scheduled.

Now this part is where I should probably not go into much detail, but I feel you should know what this entails. I had *no* idea what they were going to do. I was just told to show up for the procedure, that it usually is "not a big deal, and you can normally go back to work the same day."

Keep in mind! There are numerous ways to do biopsies; this is just one way. I have had other biopsies done differently. Please ask about your procedure, what it entails, and what you should be prepared for.

I showed up and was promptly escorted back to the room where the procedure would be done. The table was set up and looked comfy except there was a hole in the table that was, ummm, just about the size of where a *boob* might fit! I was thinking, *That looks interesting.* The nurse said, "Have you had one of these done before [like an oil change or something]?" I said, "No." She then started to explain rather quickly what they would be doing.

I was still looking at the hole in the table. It was interesting. I was thinking, *Where do they get these tables? What if it was my other boob? Is there a hole on the other side too?* So I probably missed out on all the information she was giving me *so quickly.*

Although I have nothing but respect and gratitude for the medical system, I think they become a little numb to these procedures. They forget that we don't have *any* idea what they are doing!

She placed me on the table, laying me on my stomach, and my left breast fell in the hole. So if you were to come into the room, you would see my booty in the air and my booby facing the floor! Now we waited for the doctor. He explained that he would numb the area where the "suspicious" lump is located; they can use the mammogram and x-ray machine to help them pinpoint exact locations. I'm OK with needles. I have had many surgeries, but if you have a needle phobia, beware.

At this point, I was face-to-face with the nurse, and the doctor was off to my side. I could also see what looked like the part one pulls out of a vacuum that collects dirt; it was hooked up to something that was hooked up to something that was all a part of this process.

They began. He gave me the shot. Ouchie. If you are sensitive to shots, I'm not going to lie to you; it stings. I mean you *are* getting a shot in your breast. But that beats what you *might* feel if you don't get it! As what they do next is make a little incision in which to insert a tiny tube that has a snipper on the end of it to snatch a piece of the tumor for pathology to do their thing with.

I was watching the nurse's face; she seemed to be frowning more than smiling. (I was not taking great comfort in this.) She was shaking her head a lot. She was using quite a bit of gauze. He was asking her, "Did ya get it?" She just kept shaking her head and saying, "I can't see. There is a lot of blood." I was looking at the vacuum cleaner, and I could see blood in it, but I figured, *Hey, must be what it's for. Better than it bleeding on the floor, right?*

They stopped several times to collect some samples on the gauze and take them into another room to get a "special x-ray" to see if they got the samples they needed.

Meanwhile, I was still laying butt up and boob down, watching the blood go through the vacuum cleaner.

They finally said they had what they needed. *Then* the doctor informed me that he *thought* he might have "nicked a blood vessel" because I was bleeding quite a bit. OK. So he was going back to the hospital now, and he was going to let the nurse stop the bleeding. *What?* OK. I mean, what do I know? She could do it, right?

She began by holding pressure on my already-torn-up boob that felt "nice"—*not!* Then she had me lift up a little bit. That was when I saw, *holy cow*, blood dripping like *crazy*. I was thinking, *This doesn't seem like a good scenario!* She then had me flip over onto my back. Made sense; should have stopped the blood flow—*for now*. She still kept pressure on it. It took some time, but she got it to slow down, then she put a butterfly stitch on it.

I asked her about the vacuum cleaner. "How much blood do you guys usually get out of one of these procedures?" She informed me, "Maybe a few drops to just barely enough to cover the bottom." Well, I had been watching the crazy thing fill up! She said, "You lost quite a bit of blood."

I told her I had planned to go back to work *because* I was told that *this* was *no big deal*. In and out. Whatever! *Please listen to me!* I am here to tell you that even if you *don't* have any difficulties, I would *not* recommend doing anything on this day. It *is* a surgical procedure. Even if you don't have this particular procedure, I have had others, and unless you are going to be fired, just go home. It really isn't worth it. Mentally and physically, this is a procedure that takes a lot out of you and can be unpredictable.

She firmly instructed me to wait in the facility for a while and to let her know if it soaked through the gauze, which it did. She changed it, and then we waited a while longer, and everything seemed to be OK. I was *not* allowed to go back to work. She was afraid any movement of that arm would start it bleeding again. She wanted me to go home and promptly get into bed and stay there and put ice packs on it.

I did exactly that. My mom was there to help me, so we just kept changing the ice packs on a regular basis. Later that evening—of course, when everyone in the house was gone except my mother and my youngest nephew, who was ten at the time—I felt something *really* cold around my breast. I thought maybe the ice pack was leaking or something. We were using those gel packs, so I wasn't sure what was going on. I gently lifted the ice pack to find that I was completely soaked in blood.

I called for my mother. I said, "I think we might have a little problem here." Then I showed her. In her words, "*Crap!*" Of course, everyone was gone! My son and my older nephew, people who could drive, were just there and had *just* left, as well as my father. My mother needed to stay with my nephew and she doesn't drive well at night, it was around 7:00 pm by now. I told her just to get me some towels and to call Dad. She did both. I was soaking through the towels *fast*. My dad got there rather quickly. I knew I needed to get to the ER, but my doctors were in the town next to us—approximately thirty minutes away where the procedure was done, which would have been ideal—or, we thought we could just go the ER in our town. I was debating on which one would be the best option. When I soaked through the second bath towel in about ten minutes' time, I knew we had to get to the closest one and go there *now*. I told Mom to give me two more towels, and off Dad and I went.

We got to the ER, and I walked in all covered in blood, but I was feeling quite fine. They were totally freaked out! "What happened to you?" one asked. I truly looked like a stab-wound victim! Someone whipped a wheelchair underneath me. I said, "Well, I am fairly certain I can walk. It just looks bad." The nurse said, "*Nope!* Not with that much blood! You gotta sit!" So they wheeled me back to get me going and into a room rather quickly. From there, things happened fast. I had lost a large amount of blood. My bra was full in both cups. My shirt and pants were soaked. I didn't realize how much I had lost. We just had to throw away my clothes. They then tried to concentrate on stopping the bleeding *by pushing very hard on my boob!* This made me feel very sick! I was feeling quite fine until they started that business! *It hurt!* I can usually take pain, and it was not too awful or bad, but I just think that I had lost so much blood that the combination wasn't so good. I started to hyperventilate. I told them I was going to pass out! They said, "It's OK. You are lying on the table. If you pass out, it's OK!" I didn't *want* to pass out. I would fight it until the end. I was feeling like I was going to throw up and pass out all at the same time, and then I *really* started hyperventilating! The doctor was trying to stop the bleeding; she was going to have to suture up the opening as she saw the blood vessel had been "nicked."

My dad had left the room because I was moaning and whimpering, and he just couldn't take it. Poor guy. Then, miraculously, another nurse appeared at the head of my bed and told me that I needed to breathe. She counted with me. She breathed with me. It was what I needed. I couldn't have gotten out of that place unless someone got me out of that place. Then she was gone once I was breathing at a normal rate, and they were done with me.

Now I just felt sick and weak. My boob wasn't feeling all that great now either! My dad had to go home to get me new clothes because we threw away *everything*. It was a long night. We were there for quite a while. Ultimately, I had a hematoma from the suture, which just means that the blood was still pooling up in there but would eventually subside. It was of concern; it had to be watched very carefully, and now that I had lost so much blood, that was of concern as well.

This was on a Monday. I would see my doctor the next day; she instructed that I could *not* go back to work. I was *so* weak. My hemoglobin levels were way down. She would see me on that Thursday anyway to discuss the biopsy and see how I was feeling.

That Thursday would be October 7, 2010. I already knew that it was cancer. They have to have proof however! My mom went back with me. My doctor first checked the hematoma. She was concerned about it and my hemoglobin count. I could tell by the way she was acting that she didn't want to tell me the results of the biopsy. She put that off until the very last.

She said, "Well, we do have the biopsy results, and it doesn't look very good, I'm afraid."

I then said, "It is cancer, huh?"

She said, "Yes."

Then she apologized, and I believe she had a few tears in her eyes; my mother had tears for sure.

I said, "Listen, no need to be upset. I knew it was even without all these tests. I could have told you it was. So what now? What do we do? What is our next step?"

She looked at me and said, "Wow, you are taking this very calmly. Are you OK?"

I said, "*Yes.* I just already knew it was. Now it's time to figure out what to do about it."

Now I can't say how other people react to this news. Everyone is different. Some are angry, scared, frustrated, "Why me?" lost, nervous, and so many more emotions. There is no right or wrong way to feel. Just feel it.

Finding out you have cancer requires you to go into a whole different realm. Your body knows it; your mind knows it. It is a battle for your survival. If you have to deal with it by calling your friends and crying, well do it! If you need to be alone, then be alone. If you need to *scream*, then *scream*! My way of dealing with it was treating it like all the other illnesses that I have had—just taking care of what needed to be taken care of.

I will tell you that the more *information* you can get the better off you will be. *Ask questions. Take another person with you at every appointment.* (Sometimes what you think you hear may not be what you heard. Two heads are better than one!) *Take notes!* Always have a notebook with you to write down information. *Ask questions, ask questions*, and *ask questions. Remember!* These guys do this same job every day, and they forget that you may not know the same things that they do. So *ask questions.* No question is a dumb one! It is your health!

Oh yeah! By the way, at this point, it occurs to me that *it is a very wise idea that you make a list of all the medications that you take. Make a list on your computer, print it out, and keep it with you always by putting it in your phone or somewhere that you have access to it because you will be asked this information frequently.*

Also, you will be asked what prior surgeries you have had, if any. All of this is great to have already put together for all your doctor appointments because trust me, they will ask!

They will also want to know what you are allergic to. Trust me, they will ask you over and over. It makes life much easier for you and them if you have the list.

Make sure to write down the name of the medication and the dosage as well as how often you take it.

Finally, I know that my story about the biopsy was incredibly long and practically everything that could have gone wrong *did*! That doesn't mean that this is going to happen to *you.* Your experience may be *much* less complicated. I just seem to be the lucky one in procedures that can have everything go wrong. I just wanted you to know the worst-case scenario, I guess, and maybe this isn't even the worst! Just focus on the facts that I started out with: how the procedure is done.

Good luck!

Chapter 2

"My Cancer Details"

I want to give you my specific information—but keep in mind that just because my cancer was a certain size or type and maybe yours isn't the same as mine—it's OK. Just use this as a reference. *Again,* I will emphasize that this is *my* information, *but* the end result is it is *cancer.* No matter how you want to look at it, it is what it is.

You can compare yours to mine and see how things look for your outcome compared to mine; it may or may not be comforting. I just want you to have the information.

If you haven't noticed by now, I just tell you how it is straight up. I don't like to sugarcoat anything. I prefer that for myself. I'm sorry if it seems a little too uncaring. I don't mean it to be. Quite the opposite. I care very much. I am with you all the way! You are not alone! Know that you *can* make it! What is in store for you will not be the funnest time in your life, but trust me, someday this will *not* be the most prominent thing.

My treatment choice was a mastectomy of the left breast. If you do not know what a mastectomy entails, let me enlighten you. I knew that my aunt had her whole breast removed and didn't choose to replace hers. I was familiar with that. Meaning, she was just flat chested on that one side, no nipple or anything. Just flat.

When a mastectomy is performed, they remove *all* the breast tissue and anything that is estrogen related. So guess what, your nipple has a *lot* to do with estrogen. Typically speaking, they make an incision, and they remove the breast tissue from inside, then they remove the nipple. They don't want anything that can have estrogen produced remaining as this is what can cause the cancer.

In my case, the skin underneath was tested and was not likely to survive the reconstruction process. Since I was already having the TRAM procedure, which I will explain in a moment, they just took a piece of skin from my stomach and transferred it to my breast.

I noticed within days after the surgery, as you will see in the photos, the triangular-shaped piece of skin. As I looked at it, I recognized the stretch marks that were on there! Hey! Those were on my stomach on the lower left side! (A girl *knows* her stretch marks!) I asked my surgeon about this at one of his visits. I said, "Am I imagining this, or is this my stomach skin? 'Cause I recognize these stretch marks!" He laughed and said, "Yes, we had to transfer that piece of skin as the remaining original skin would have died." Well *hey*, I don't remember seeing or reading anything about *that*! I told him so! He said that perhaps he forgot to go over that little detail with me. *Hmmmm.* I'm not complaining. I'm just saying it was a little surprising to find my stomach on my boob! Following along with that, my *mother* thought she might inform me one day that . . . well, she tried to be delicate, but she said, "Honey, I don't know if you've noticed, but *you have hair on your boob*!" *Gee*, thanks, Mom! Yes, I did notice it. You know the fine tiny, little hairs that are around down there! At least mine are blonde!

The TRAM procedure is where they remove fat from your stomach and transfer it to your breast. Sounds all good, huh? I am proud to say that my doctor said I only had enough fat for *one* breast. So you basically get a tummy tuck out of the deal. Still sounds good, right? Well, this is a *very* complex procedure. Not only do they transfer the fat, but they also reroute all your blood vessels from where they were before to the boob area where it is now so there is little or no chance of your body rejecting it. It is *yours*.

I chose this option for more than one reason. I have had many surgeries, and having implants requires more than one surgery usually, so I wanted the least amount of surgical procedures possible. I was at risk of rejection of the implant. There were many reasons for my decision, but this ultimately was what I chose.

If you choose this option, please note that it takes a little bit longer for recovery. The surgery isn't pretty, and you'll look like you've been hunted down and tortured by Freddy Krueger himself! *But* in the end, I have a very natural-looking result. You must choose what is right for you.

Let me talk about losing one's nipple for a moment. It is a *huge* thing right now. I know that it seems like a totally bizarre scenario. Maybe your spouse/loved one is freaked out about it too. Sometimes it is difficult to even bring the subject up. But, THIS, THIS IS WHY I HAVE GIVEN YOU THIS TOOL. I want you to know that even though things are going to change with your body, it doesn't mean that you can't have a relationship with your loved one. It *is* going to look different, but let's compare *cancer vs. nipple*. Trust me, you can live without your nipple. I have found that there are several advantages to it:

1. I only "nip out" on one side.
2. It makes a good party topic.
3. If you wear a padded bra, you can make people guess which one is real.

Finally, at my house, I refer to my breast as my Belly Boob. You must laugh at yourself some! It really does help.

Now after all is said and done, you *can* have a nipple back, if you want. Your plastic surgeon will discuss your options. You can have an "outy" all the time, or you can have a tattoo. I chose to have the tattoo. The outy is another small surgical procedure.

Please, please, please, now—right now—look up the closest cancer-care organization. If you don't know how, look up American Cancer Society in your phone book or google it. They will direct you to the correct organization. *You need stuff!* You will need things that you don't even *know* you need! They will have garments that you can wear after your surgery that will help hold the drains. They have *comfort pillows*, or at least, I hope they do for you. Your arm will be sore, and these pillows are awesome. They also have wigs and scarves, as well as nutrition supplements.

I was *not* aware of this until *way* after my surgery. They gave me the comfort pillows, and I *still* use them sometimes, and how *I wish I had them long before then.*

Enough about that. I know you may want to know more about my specific type of cancer. There is a lot of information that I truly don't remember. So I asked my oncologist for a summary of my cancer and treatment. If you are going through breast cancer and you have a pathology report, the following information will make some sense to you. You are flooded with information right now, and hopefully, some of it is making some sense to you. If it isn't, *ask questions, lots and lots of questions.* You can't find out the answers if you don't ask the questions.

The problem is that sometimes we don't know what questions to ask. *So* have faith in your doctors. If you don't have a good relationship with your doctor, *change doctors.* It is crucial to have a good relationship with your doctor. *Do the best thing for your life! It is your health. It is your survival on the line.*

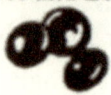
July 12, 2012

Conway, Dana

Dx: Breast cancer – invasive ductal – Stage IC; ER+, PR-, Her-2 0
Tx: Left breast mastectomy with SLN bx, no XRT; TC x4 – 1ˢᵗ cycle 1/4/11, 2ⁿᵈ cycle 1/25/11, 3ʳᵈ cycle 2/15/11, 4ᵗʰ cycle 3/8/11; Femara 2.5mg qd started 3/29/11 (surgical menopause) x5 yrs

One History: In review, she has Stage IC invasive ductal left breast cancer. She had menarche at age 13, G4P1 – one son (age 28 at 1ˢᵗ pregnancy), surgical menopause at age 40 with TAH-BSO (done due to endometriosis, h/o ectopic pregnancy x2, menorrhagia). On HRT from 2005 thru 10/2010. Prior left breast biopsy on 8/26/06 – pathology showed fibrocystic changes. She has +FH for cancers – MGF kidney cancer, MGM "unknown cancer to the bones", 1 aunt with breast cancer, 2ⁿᵈ aunt with "GYN cancer", no other definite cancers in the family. BRCA screening on 10/26/10 was negative. She had normal bilateral screening mammography on 7/2/10. In late 9/2010 she noted some fullness in the upper inner quadrant of her left breast and subsequent diagnostic left breast mammography on 9/28/10 showed two areas of microcalcifications at 10 o'clock measuring 1.2x0.5cm; US left breast on 9/28/10 confirmed a 0.5cm area of concern at 10 o'clock. She had left breast biopsy on 10/4/10 – pathology showed invasive ductal carcinoma (2/8 cores, 0.2cm, grade 3) and adjacent extensive DCIS (grade 3, solid/comedo types). ER 96%/PR 0%/Ki-67 45%/Her-2 0. She had L breast mastectomy + SLN bx with immediate reconstruction on 11/12/10. Final pathology showed an invasive ductal carcinoma (grade 2, 1.8cm, 0/2 LNs, clear margins, +LVI) with associated DCIS (solid + comedo, grade 3) – staged as pT1cpN0M0 or Stage IC. There is no role for radiation. Labs from 10/14/10 – WBC 5.2, Hgb 10.6, Plt 354, CMP normal. She had CT A/P on 10/4/10 for abdominal pain – showed hepatic cyst/hemiangioma in the liver, left kidney stone, but was otherwise normal.CXR on 5/19/10 was normal. MRI Brain 5/25/10 was essentially normal, possible sinusitis. There is no indication to obtain additional screening studies like repeat CT A/P, bone scan, CXR, etc. Oncotype DX for further risk stratification had RS of 29 (intermediate risk, 19% recurrence @ 5 yrs with Tamoxifen alone); she has chosen to have TC x4cycles (1ˢᵗ cycle 1/4/11, 2ⁿᵈ cycle 1/25/11, 3ʳᵈ cycle 2/15/11, 4ᵗʰ cycle 3/8/11) followed by AI x5 years. She reported syncopal episode – referred to CV – dx with neurocardiogenic syncope, no specific tx recs. US LLE on 1/25/11 (for LLE pain) showed no DVT and reduction of L saphenous vein thrombosis. CT A/P on 1/25/11 (for LLQ pain) showed no acute abnormalities. She has seen Dr. Storm for small incisional fluid collection; no I&D planned, finished 10d course of Levaquin in 2/2011. Bone density scan 3/30/11 showed osteopenia of the B femurs but normal LSpine. R breast mammogram 5/20/11 showed stable calcs @superior medial R breast. CBE with Dr. Paulsen on 5/24/11 normal. Had been seeing Dr. Storm for L breast chest wall wound from prior surgery – fully healed as of 11/2011. Had fall on 10/13/11 – apparent possible hairline fracture of R ankle; following with Podiatry and was wearing a "boot" for some time.

Chapter 3

"Surgery"

S*o* I almost did what I have accused the medical profession of doing! I almost left this chapter completely out! I just assumed that all of you have had *twenty surgeries like me*!

Seriously, I have had twenty surgeries. They have become rather routine for me. I realize now that I should help you with some information about what to expect when you go in for your surgery. No matter what surgery you have, you can expect something in the nature of what I am about to tell you.

First of all, *it is OK to be scared*. I am always nervous before a surgery. I was particularly nervous before this one, and it was important to me to have family there for this surgery. Most of the time, I'm OK if you just drop me off and show up after it's all done. That doesn't mean that I wasn't nervous for the other surgeries, there was just a sense of anxiety that I had never felt before. I tried to rationalize it by the fact that it was Cancer, but really it wasn't that. I just couldn't put my finger on it. Like I said, I have had quite a few surgeries, so I just know what to expect.

So what does happen?
Well, normally, they have you fast the night before—from midnight on. No drinking or eating after midnight. They will have you stop some medications up to a week prior to your surgery. The hospital's

surgical nurse should call you to go over all the details approximately a week before your surgery. Remember the list I was telling you about? The list of your medications and such? Have it ready! They go over it!

The morning of or day of your surgery, they usually ask you to be there about two hours before your surgery's scheduled time. Sometimes they will ask you to not wear any fingernail polish and have absolutely *no* makeup. (I have tried to sneak in the makeup part. No go. They always make me wash it off.) I have gotten away with the fingernail polish though.

When you arrive, they will check you in, they will weigh you, and they will check your vitals (blood pressure, pulse, temperature). They normally allow you to have at least one person go back with you. *Again*, that list—your meds, surgeries, etc.—they will want to go over *all* of that again. They will ask you what you are in there for *a lot*.

You will have to take all your clothes off, and I mean all. I usually come in wearing something loose fitting. I would suggest that you wear something that zips up the front; it will be a *lot* easier to get back on when you leave. I usually wear sweats or something easy to get on or off. Remember, you are not there for a fashion show. You won't be wearing these clothes long. I would also suggest wearing slip-on shoes—nothing that you have to tie up; bending over will not be fun. *Simple, simple, simple.*

You will have to take your clothes off and put on one of their fashionable hospital gowns, and they usually give you some warm booties for your feet. (I have a rather-large collection of hospital booties.) Then they will cover you up with a nice heated blanket! That is always good!

Next, they will probably start an IV. Most of the time, they will put it on the opposite arm of where they are working. Sometimes they have to put more than one in. It depends on your situation. If you have never had an IV started before, it may seem scary to you. I will tell you that it really isn't that bad. These nurses do this *all* the time, and they are well trained in their job, so *trust them. Relax*, it is crucial to them to be able to find a vein. This is what they are doing. They are starting a direct line into your vein so that they can put medicine directly into your bloodstream. So the needle is directly put into your vein, and then, there is a little plastic tube that is left behind. Then you will see on the surface, there is a tube-looking contraption, and it has a cap on it. More than likely, they will start you on just a normal saline solution to start hydrating you. They will numb you with a little shot in the area where they are trying to start the IV, and yes, it stings a little bit, but it isn't horrible. You will feel pressure where they put the needle in the vein, but it shouldn't be painful. After this part, you are home free. All the medicines can be given to you through this.

So now you are all ready to wait! You will have to wait for your surgeon and the anesthesiologist and possibly your plastic surgeon.

You will not go back for surgery until you have talked to all of them. They will go over the procedures again with you. If you have *any questions, now is the time to ask. Don't be afraid! Ask! Ask! Ask!*

If you feel like crying, cry. If you just want to be alone, be alone. If you need to pray, pray. But trust me, you will be fine. Because the next thing that comes your way, you are going to like!

Once you are all secure with what the doctors are going to do, they will get ready to take you back. They will give you this *lovely medicine* called Versed. I call it my margarita! It makes you very happy! From here on, you just won't care what goes on!

Now before all this goes on, before you go back, they will talk to you about pain levels. If you are in pain right now, how much, etc. They will try to make you give it a number—rating your pain from 1 to 10, with 1 being the lowest and 10 being the highest. This gives them a base level of how much pain you are in right now compared to how much pain you might be in after surgery.

OK, let's be clear. *Don't be afraid of the pain. I know; easy for me to say. Well, I have been there, and you can do it!* You may have a high tolerance for pain; you may have a low tolerance for pain. It doesn't matter. When you go back for surgery, just know in your mind that you *might* have some pain. *Don't be afraid to tell the nurse that you are in pain, and if in doubt as to what number to tell them, you should tell them you are hurting, and they will take it from there.*

Now for me, I always tell them it's 8 unless I have no pain at all. If I'm hurting, it's an 8 or a 10. I have a fairly high tolerance for pain. Here is the key; it is *crucial*! If the nurses are going to be able to do their job, and that is to control your pain, they can't do it if you don't *tell* them you are in pain! Controlling your pain starts with you telling them you are in pain. They can continue keeping you *out* of pain from that point on.

I got a little out of sequence here. They will wake you up from your nice lullaby sleep. You will be in the nicest sleep you have ever had. Nurses all have their ways of waking you, but it is never fun because you are in this nice, peaceful sleep, then you have someone calling your name, waking you up! Generally, this is *very* startling! It's OK to feel that way. The nurses are trained to handle this. This is when they will start asking you about the pain.

Again, everyone reacts to surgery differently. The anesthesia can make you feel sick. This is normal. If you start feeling sick when you are waking up, *call the nurse.* They have medicine for that.

I tend to get migraines after I wake up from the anesthesia, so I take my prescription migraine medicine with me, and they know to give it to me if I start complaining about a headache.

From this point on, you will be in the care of mostly your nurses. I highly recommend that you be congenial to them! They are much nicer to you if you are cordial to them and thank them for things. They have a job to do, and they can do it well. Like all of us, we'd rather take care of people who are nice to us and will most likely go the extra mile for such people.

One other thing is that you might have to go on a blood thinner. Some might have to administer shots in your stomach. If you do, *do not be afraid*. This is not a big deal. I was terrified to do this. However, the needle is *so small*, and it is automated, and it literally takes seconds and doesn't hurt. (Well, maybe just a little, but not much.) I would say it hurts more *after* you have the shot, when the medicine is in. You *need to do this*. You do *not* want a blood clot, especially after you have gone through all of this. So you got to do this! *You can!* You will be shown how. It is quick and easy. You just pinch an area of fat on your stomach and poke the needle in and inject. It's really fast!

I promise you, *you can do this*!

I hope I didn't scare you. I want to *inform*! *I'm cheering you on!*

Chapter 4

"Pictures of My Progression"

Let me begin by telling you that for some reason, maybe just my own curiosity, I began taking pictures of myself from the day before my surgery to postsurgery and to my progression thereafter. Most of the pictures I have were taken with my iPhone. I took them myself as I was healing; it's kind of hard to find someone to snap naked photos of you!

When I found that I had cancer and I chose to have a mastectomy, the question lying heavily on my mind was "What am I going to look like?" I wanted to know what was in store for me.

I did my research, but what I found was just before and after pictures. My particular procedure choice was to have a full mastectomy of the left breast with a TRAM reconstruction and reconstruction and lift of the right breast.

A TRAM procedure involves removing the fat from the stomach and transferring it to the breast. Basically, you get a tummy tuck sort of a thing. Sounds great, right? Well, not as easy as it seems. The incision in the stomach is from hip to hip, and there are drainage tubes that are in place, so that is some of what you will see. They did take four lymph nodes, there is an extra incision up near my armpit for that, and they had to transfer skin from my stomach to my breast. So when you see the pictures, you will notice that there is a triangular-shaped piece on there. Also, they had to make me a new belly button as my old one was discarded when the skin was pulled down. This procedure is very intricate and involved; they not only transfer the fat, but they also reroute all the blood vessels and veins to the fat so there is little or no chance of rejection.

I still have no feeling in my breast and most of my trunk area. The nerve endings were damaged. They may eventually come back, and I think that I have slowly gotten feeling back in some areas.

Having said all of that, I want you to know that these pictures are graphic. I *wanted* them for reference, and if you choose to skip over some of the surgical ones, I understand. Again, let me remind you that these are *my* results. Your results will be *your* results. However, I hope this helps you to know what the possible outcome might be.

This first picture was taken the day before my surgery.

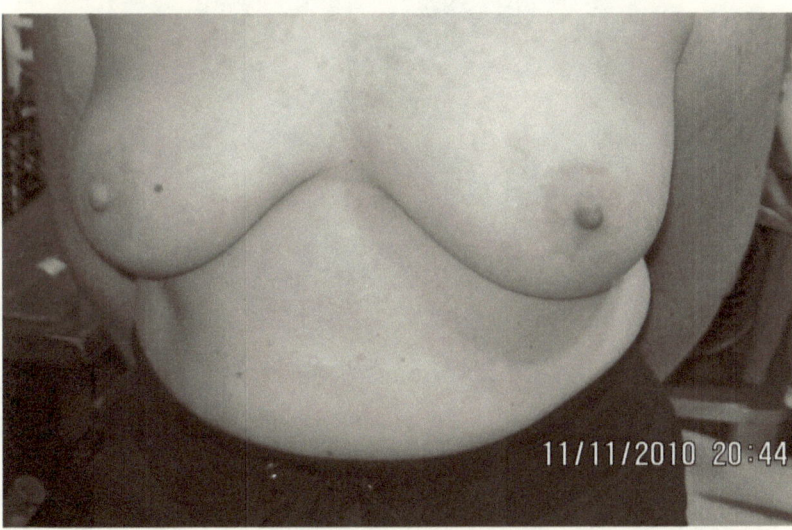

These next pictures were taken after I returned home from the hospital. Let me tell you, when I looked at myself at this point, I was trying to figure out how in the world this was ever going to look like a boob!

There were drains that had to be stripped and emptied twice daily. I must say that this part was the only really painful part. They have to suture the drains to your skin, so when the tubes are pulled on, it pulls on the skin, and the drains are so deep inside it really is just uncomfortable. But it's not the most horrible pain I've ever been in. (I compare everything to labor!)

I will just post them in the order I took them that day. Also, you will notice my belly button in several of them. They had to make a new one. It looked horrible, like a huge spider had landed in there. This also required special care. Just remember that these are all postsurgery pictures.

I want to thank my best friend, Cheryl Krug-Laskey, for taking these for me! I insisted that we take them. It was shocking for her to see this horrible mess, but she is a true friend! She was a trooper! Thanks, girlfriend!

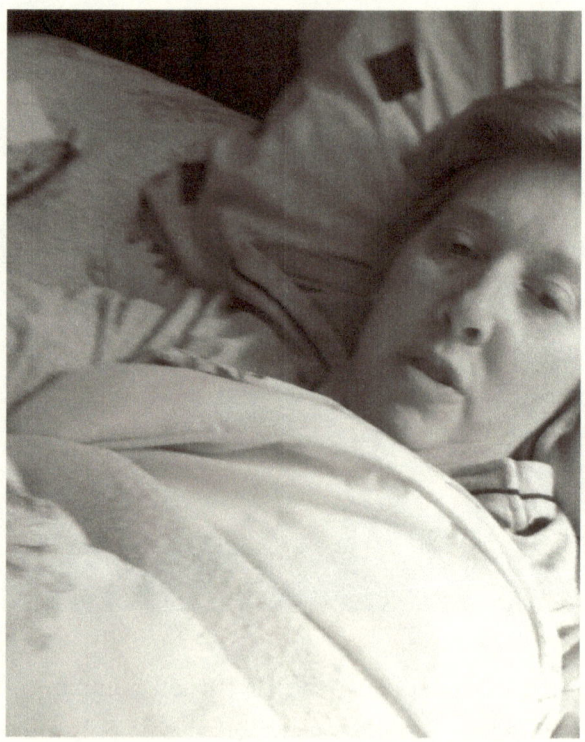

This was my position for quite a long time! Lying here in bed!

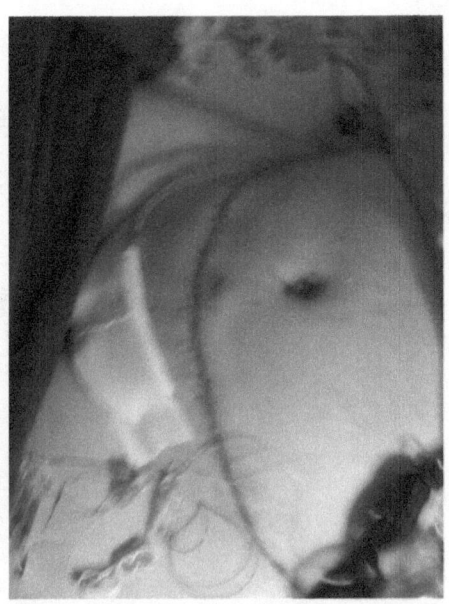

November 17, 2010
(All the following pictures are of the same
date until you see a different one.)

You will notice in these pictures the incision I was talking
about as well as the drains and my lovely belly button.

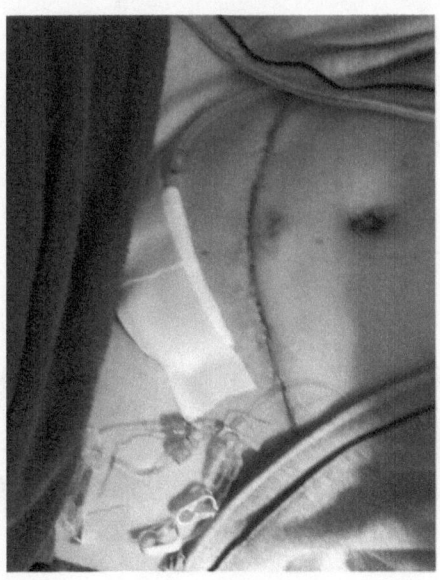

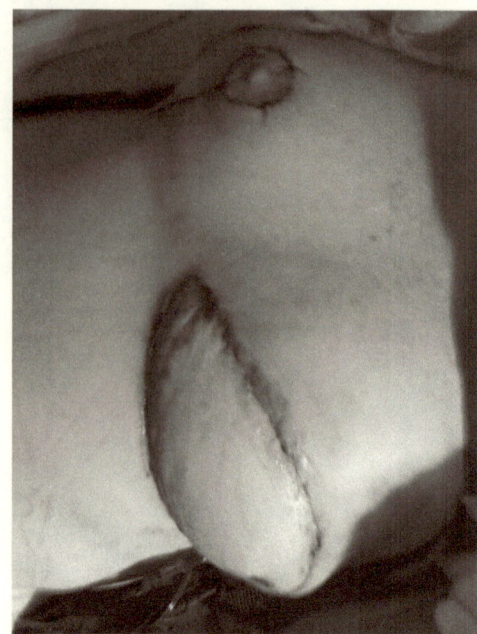

In these next few pictures, you will notice the
drainage tube just below the breast.

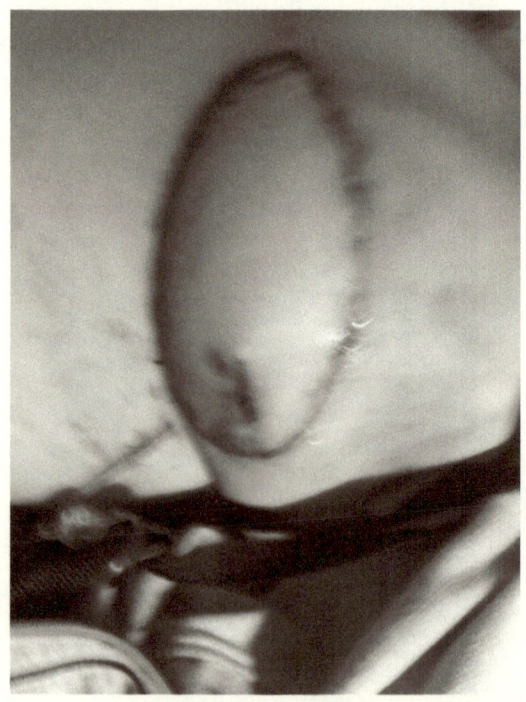

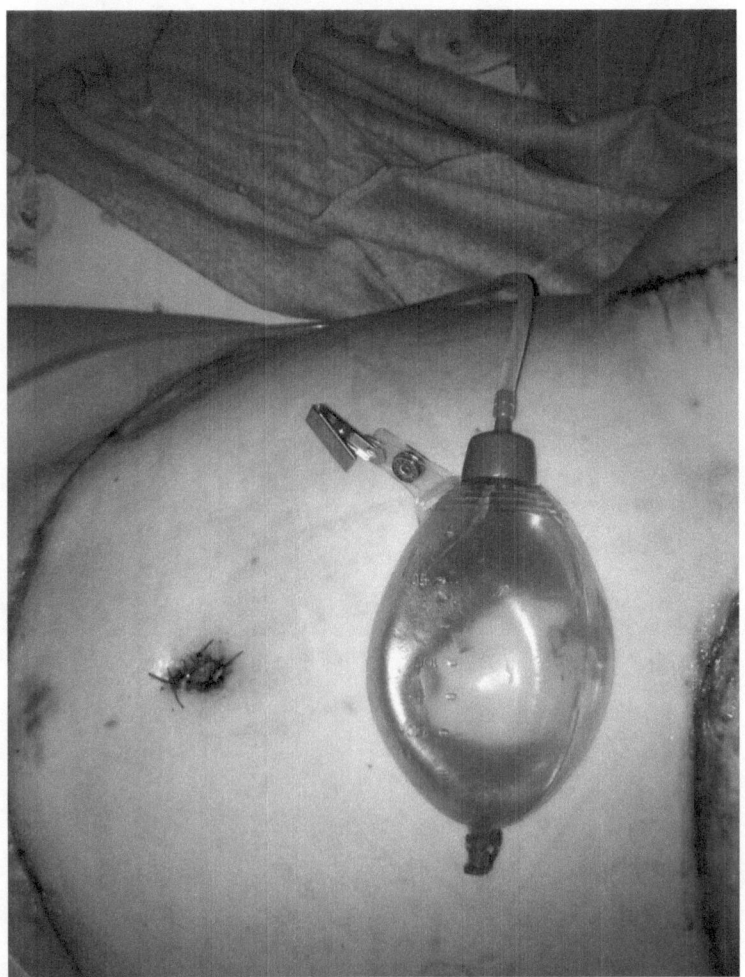

This bulb is where the fluid drains to. This is the drainage tube from my lower abdomen. The stripping that I spoke of required squeezing or pinching off the tube at the base and pulling the fluid down to the bulb. Then we would have to measure it and discard it. The blue tip just flips open to drain the fluid out. You can see that there is a small clip; that is to clip to your clothes. I would recommend that you contact someone at the American Cancer Society; they can direct you to a local establishment. They have these *great* garments that have compartments that these fit in! (I wasn't aware that there was such a thing until after.)

This next set of pictures shows the progress after the surgery.

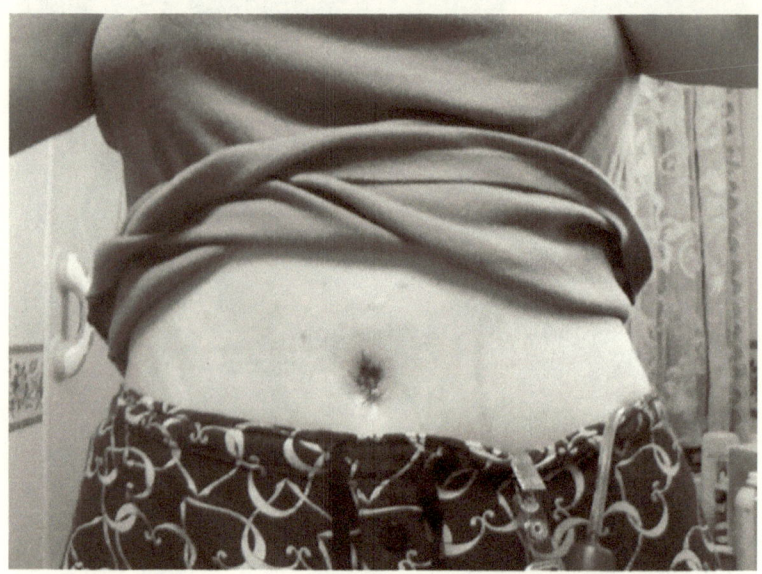

If you notice, the clip I was referring to is on my pants, and the drain is hanging here. I believe this is about one week out from surgery. November 20, 2010.

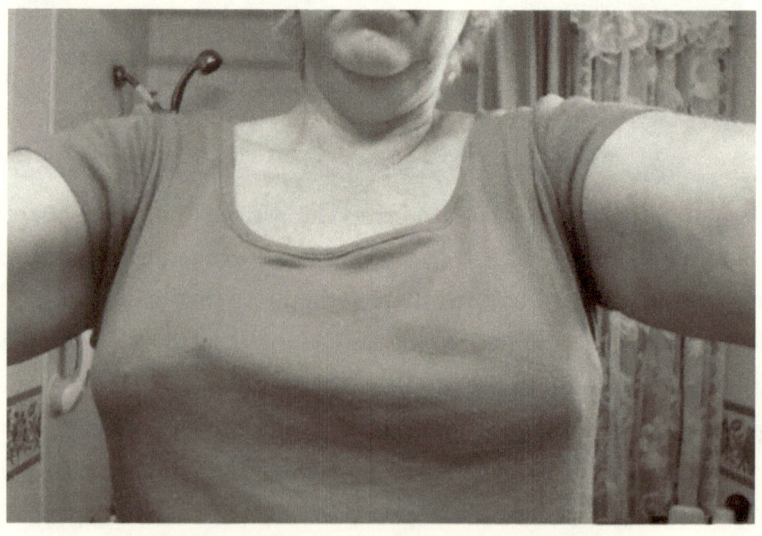

Taken the same day as the previous picture.
I believe there is still one drain in my breast, but it's not too bad for one week out! November 20, 2010.

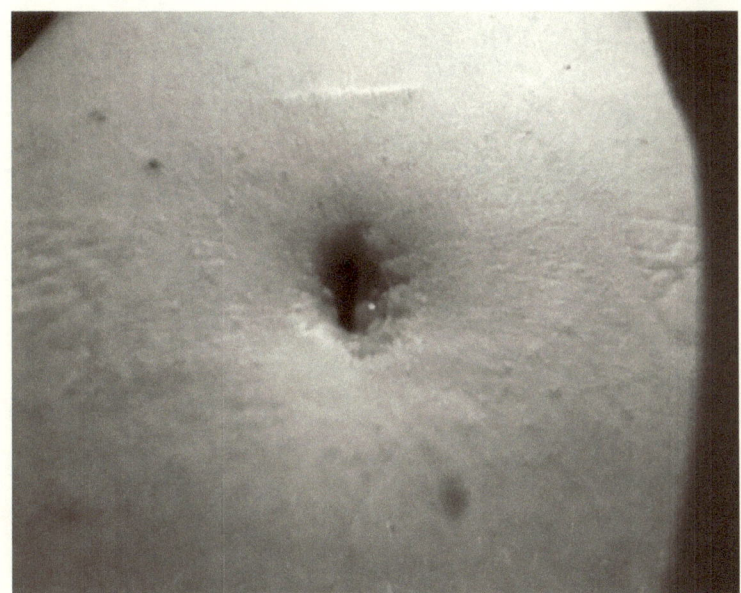

As you can see, the sutures have been removed, and I have a belly button, but it took a *long* time to heal. I had to treat it with antibiotic cream for quite a while. December 8, 2010.

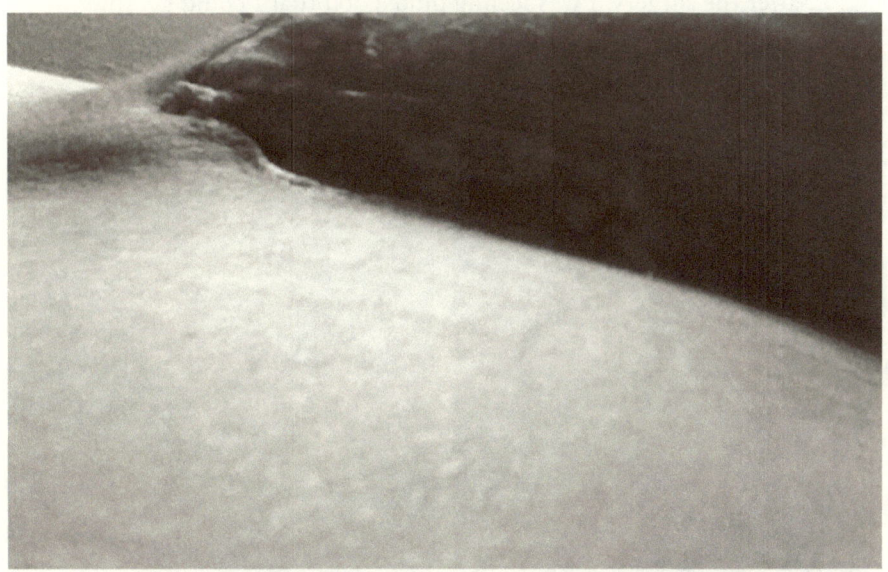

This area was difficult. It is underneath the left breast. It took a *long* time to heal and also required some antibiotic ointment. December 8, 2010.

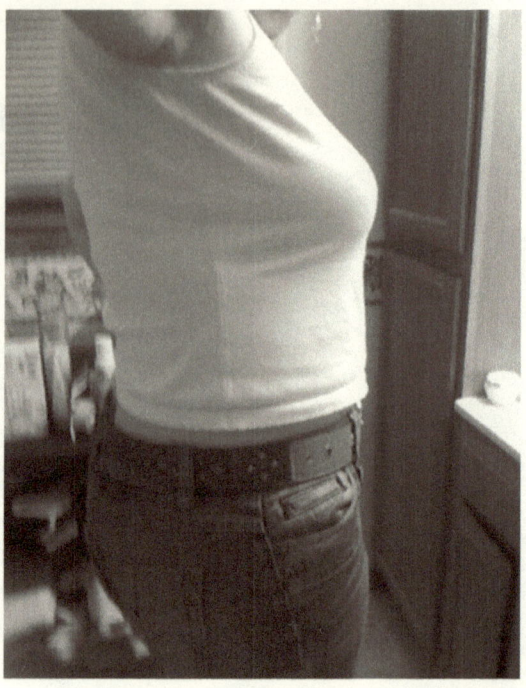

These next few pictures were taken approximately one month after the surgery. I was feeling quite good that I could get into these jeans. (I didn't wear them for long. I was still swollen and a bit sore from the surgery.) December 10, 2010.

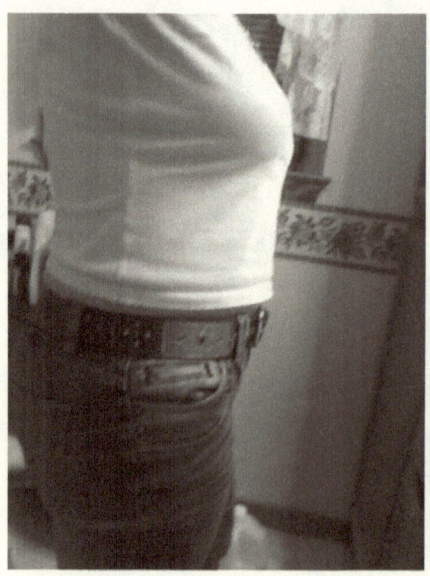
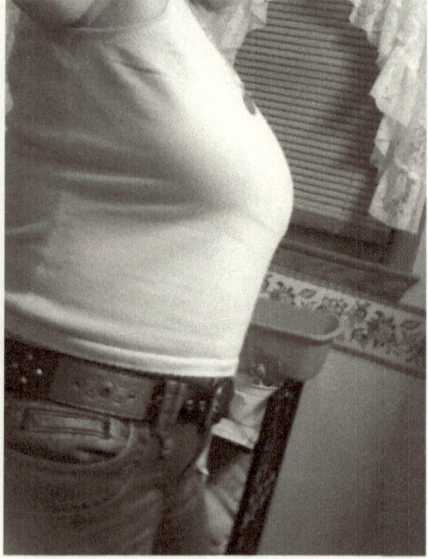

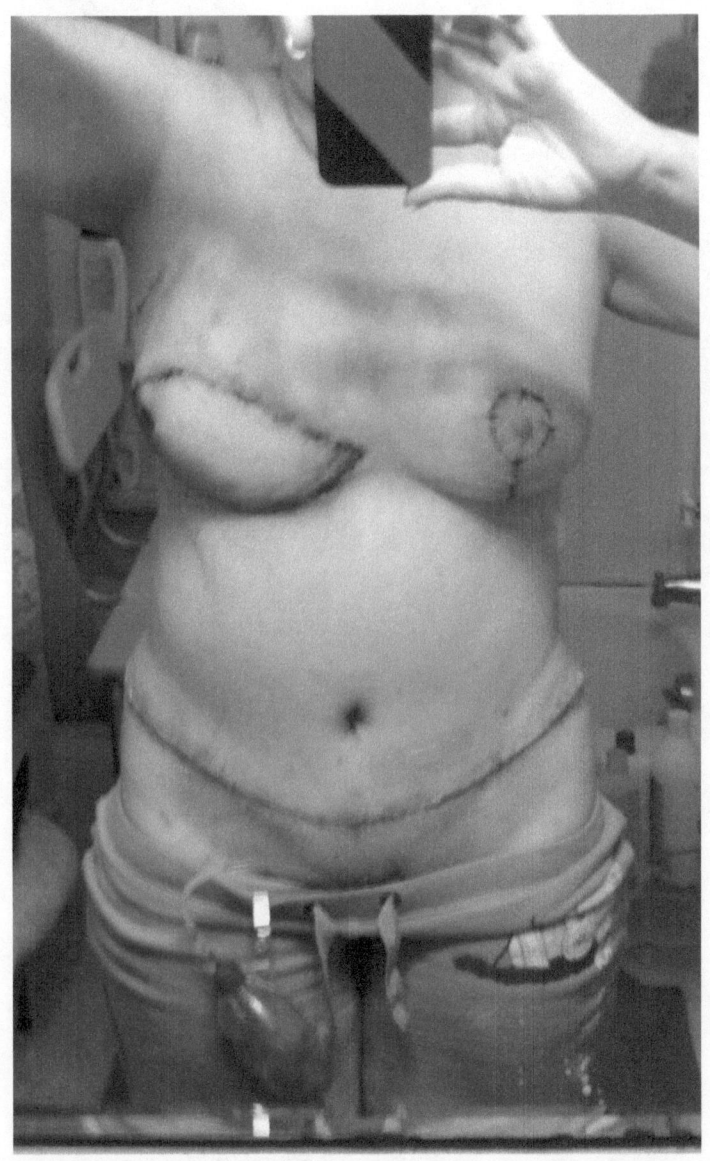

November 20, 2010. *Remember, these pics were taken in a mirror!*
So my left breast is flipped! You will see when you look at the final
pictures taken with a camera and the direct pictures previously taken.

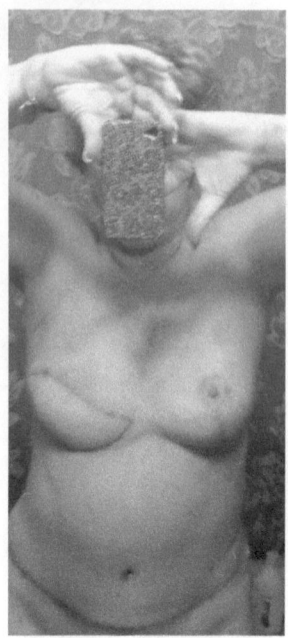

March 15, 2011

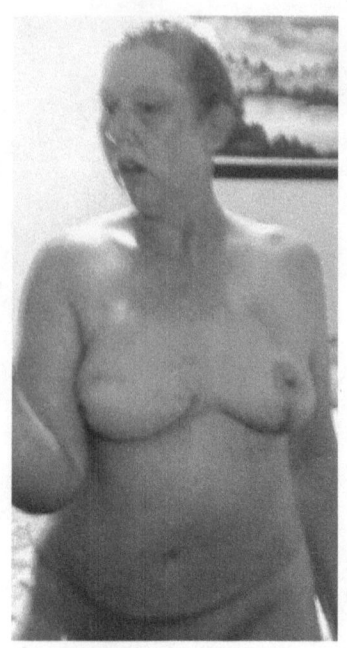

July 16, 2011

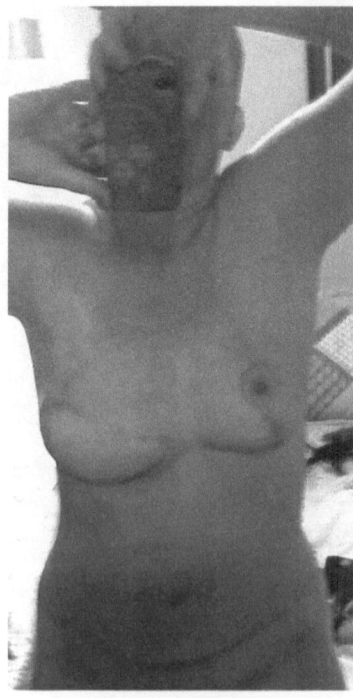

July 16, 2011

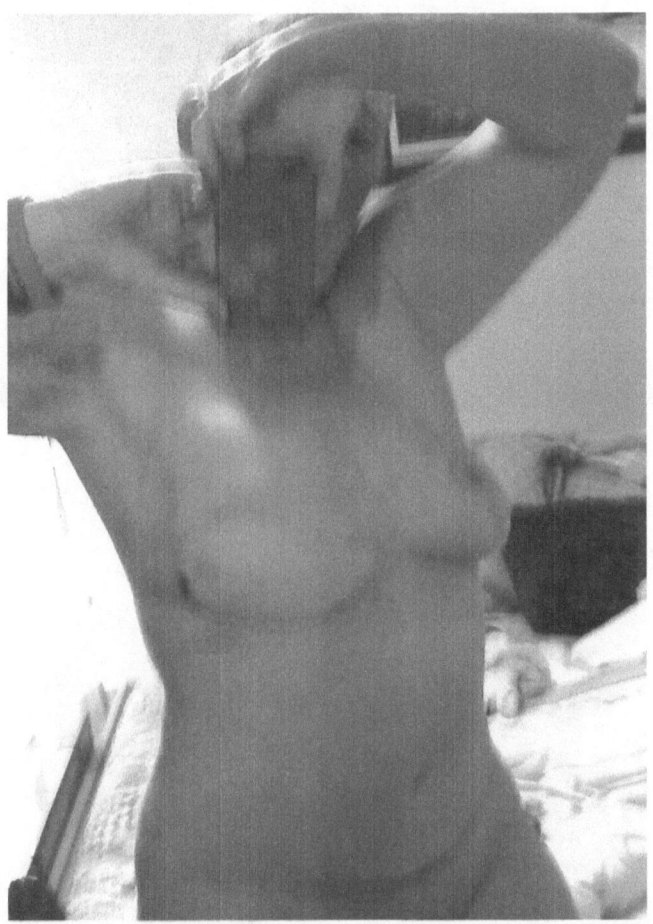

If you notice in this picture, you'll see that there is a dark area on the right breast (remember, these are taken in a mirror, so they are reversed. It's actually on the left side of this picture). This was an open wound that was not healed from a surgery I had a few months back; the surgery was to remove some scar tissue that had formed from the reconstruction. We had to clean out and pack this wound for almost four weeks. The wound was almost five centimeters deep and the size of a nickel wide. But it finally healed. (Picture taken on July 16, 2011.)

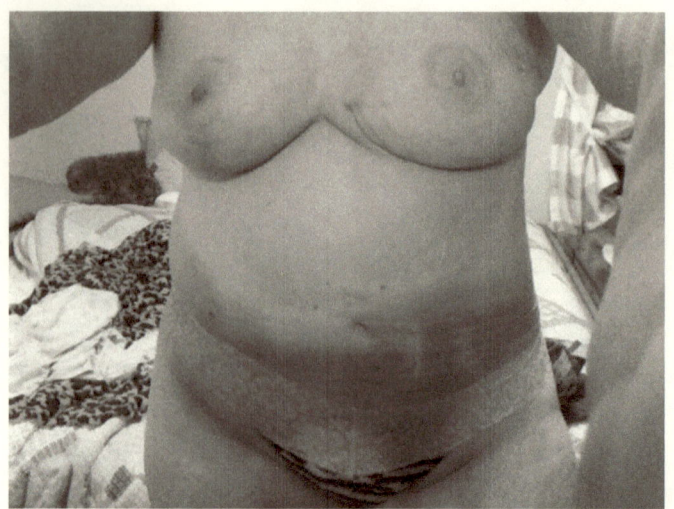

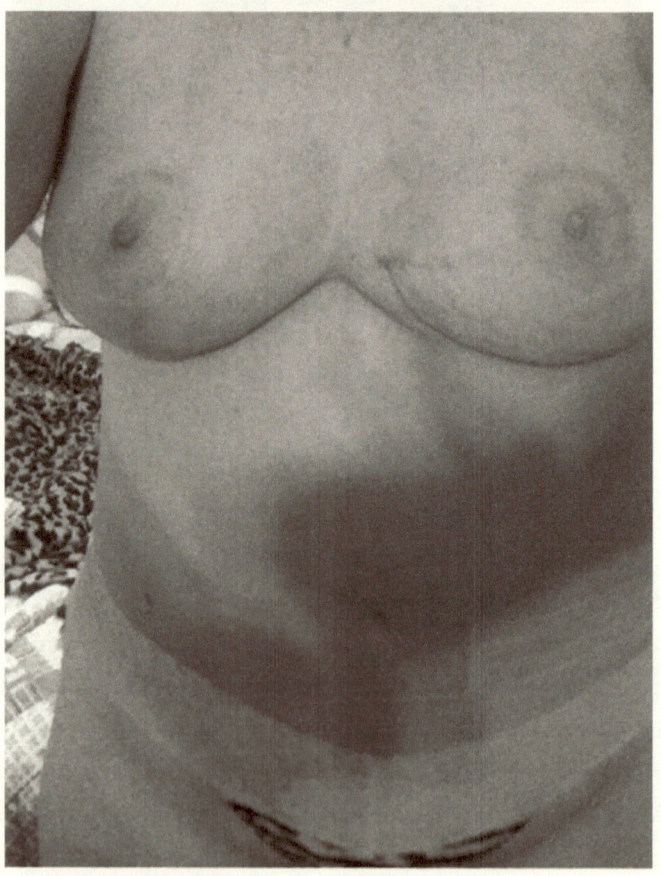

March 29, 2012

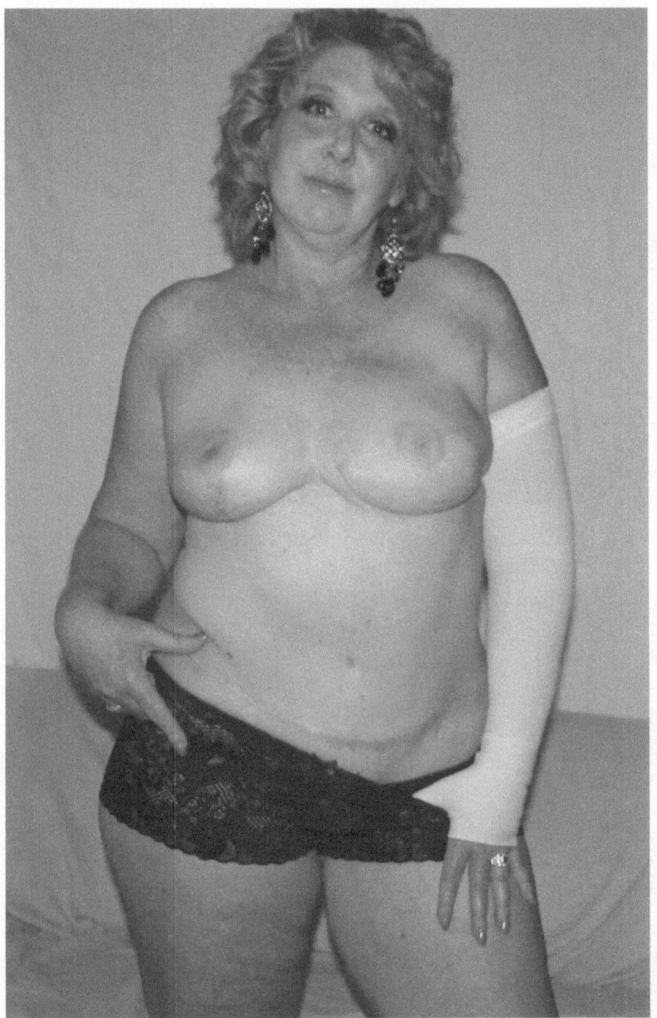

August 12, 2012

(These next pictures were taken last year by my niece Ashley Conway.)
By the way, notice the pink sleeve/gauntlet. If you don't know
what these are by now, you *need* to have a talk with your physician.
All breast-cancer survivors with any lymph-node removal are at
risk for lymphedema. You should have had physical therapy, and
you should have received a fitting for a compression sleeve.

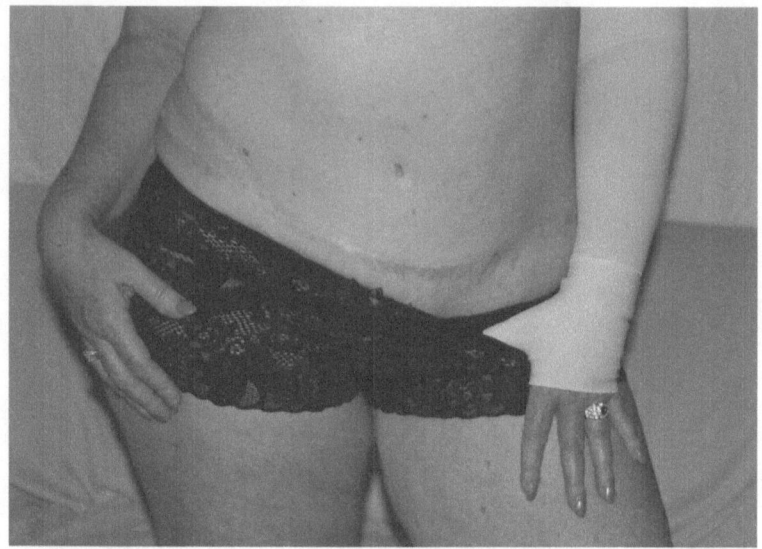

August 12, 2012. Here I am showing the healing of the abdomen scar.

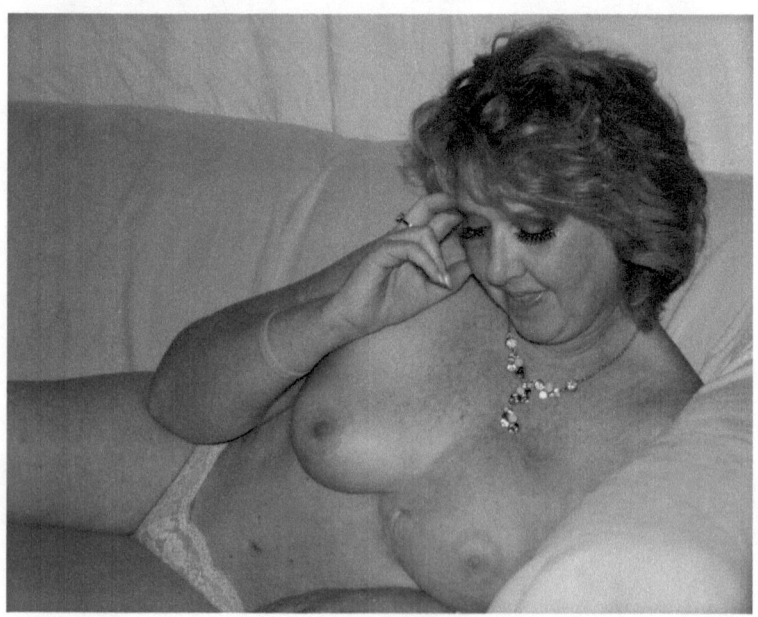

August 12, 2012

As you notice, I have had my breast tattoo. It is not exactly like the right one, yet still convincing. If you look real close at the left one, you can still see a small scar real close to the cleavage.

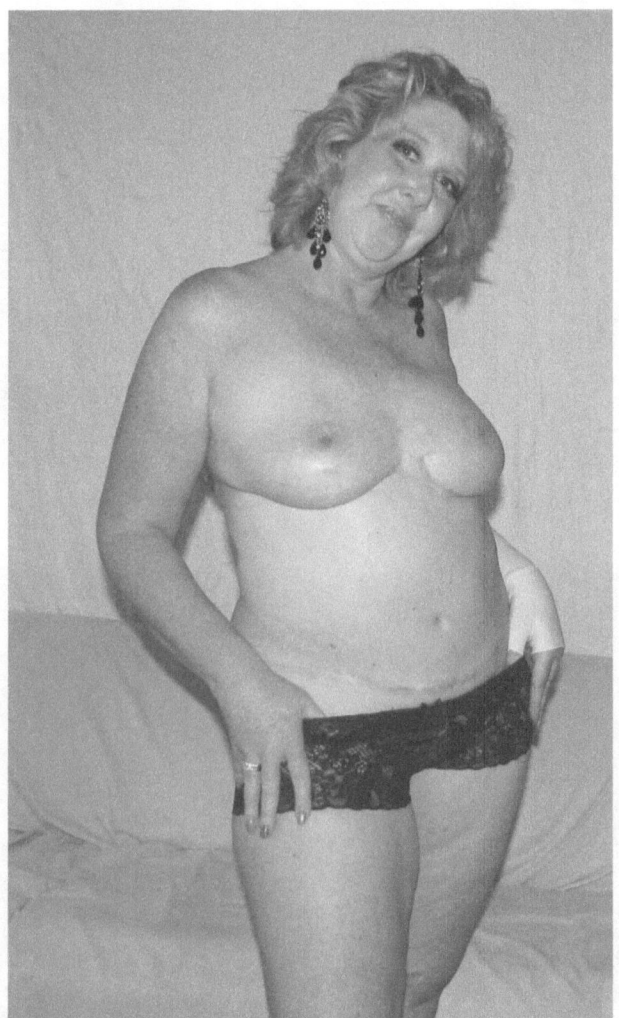

August 12, 2012. Remember, the right breast was reconstructed
as well. You can see it looks OK. You can see that scar on
the left breast here. This was the hard-to-heal area.

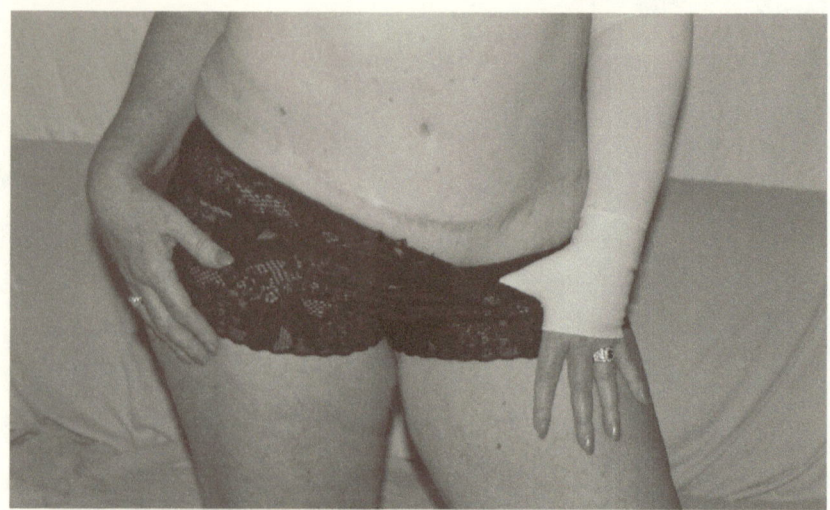

August 12, 2012. My itty-bitty belly button.

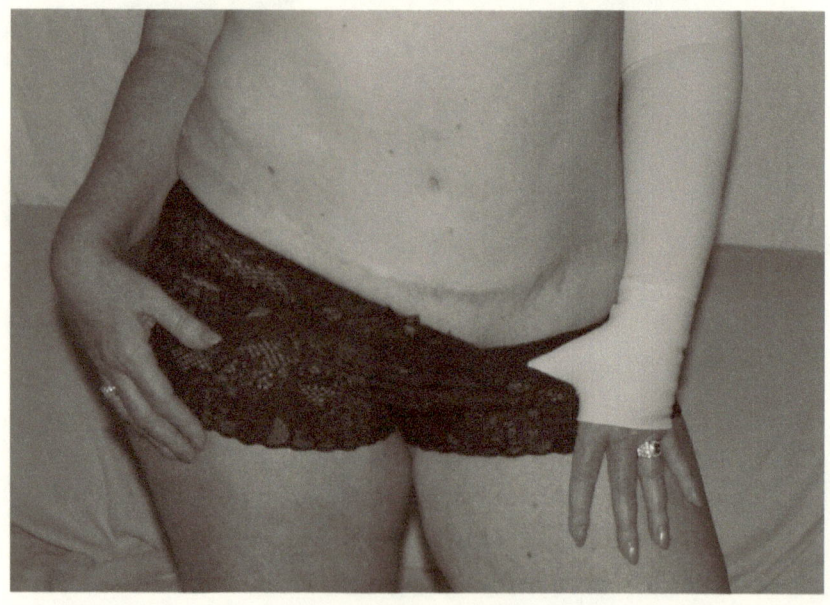

August 12, 2012

You can see the area right in the middle has a deeper scar. I
had a second surgery to remove some scar tissue there.

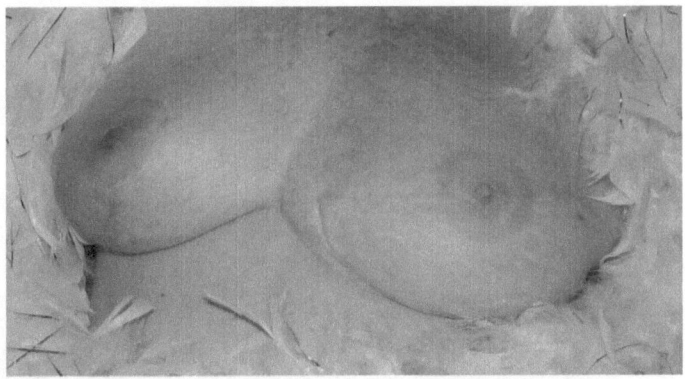

August 12, 2012. In this photo, you can really see my description of the stretch marks that was on my stomach. Remember, this skin was from my abdomen and transplanted up here. You can just barely see the scar going across now where the two pieces were attached.

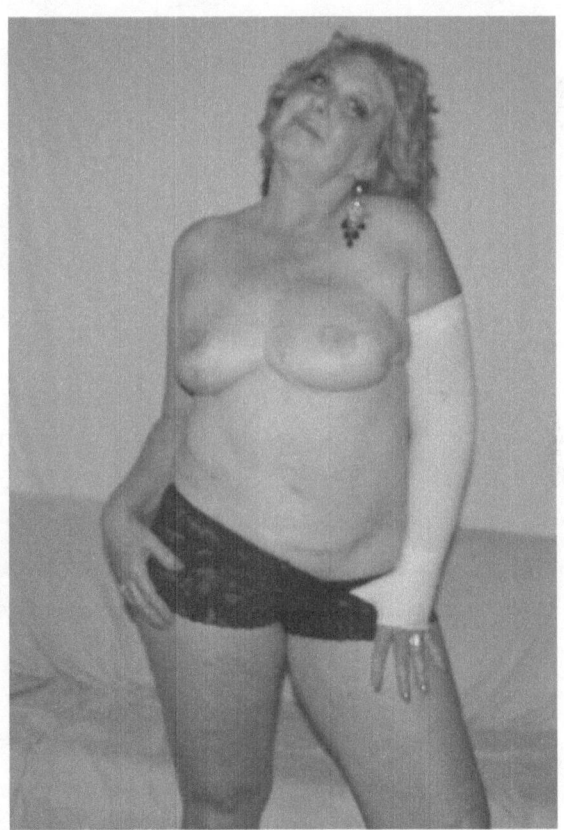

August 12, 2012. Like I said, I just want you to see that it can be OK.

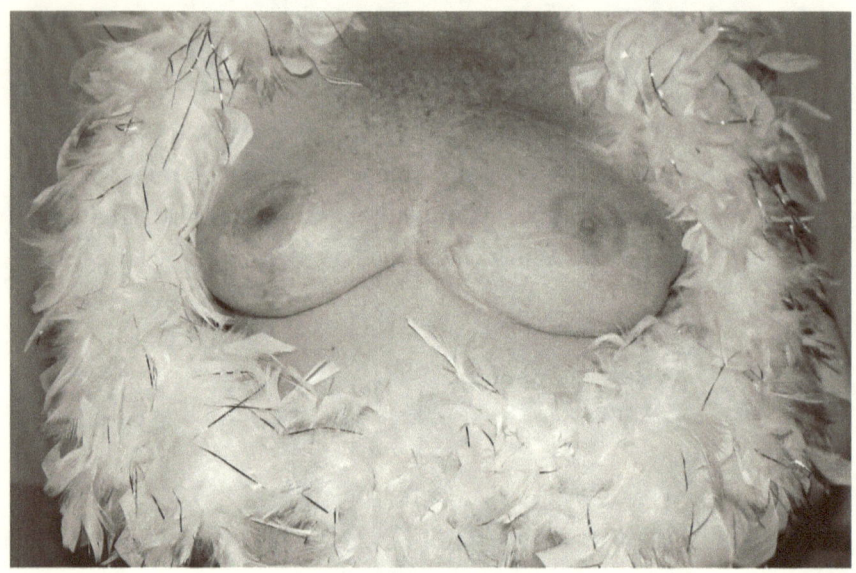

August 12, 2012

(If you will notice, there are stretch marks on the breast on your right, which is actually my left breast and the one with the reconstruction. You will also notice the nipple tattoo.) The stretch marks are from the skin that was removed from my abdomen during the reconstruction. But if you flip back to the original pictures, you will see that it looks *much* more like a breast than what I started with.

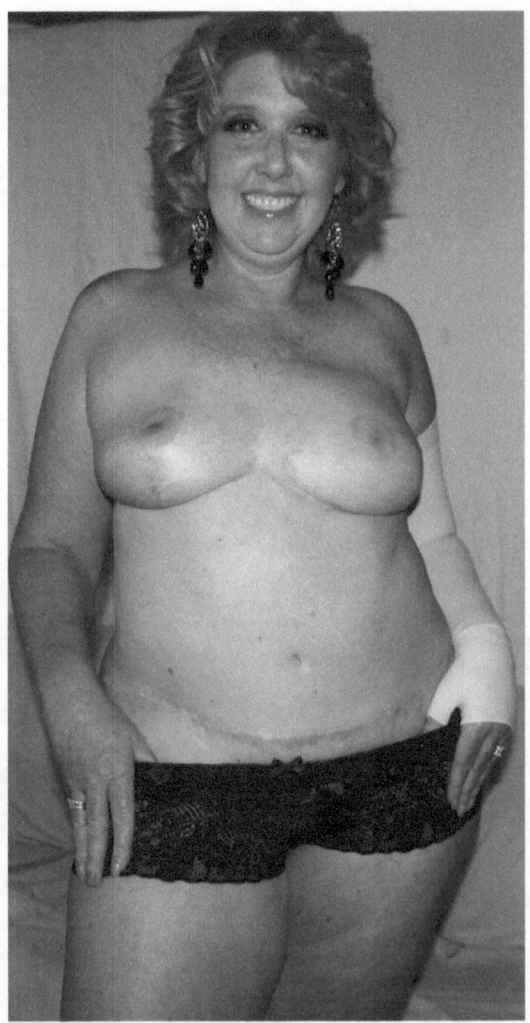

In these pictures, I wanted to make sure that you are seeing the scar
has healed fairly well along my abdomen. With the exception of
right at the center area, where it is still a little raised due to another
follow-up surgery, the rest of the area has healed quite nicely.

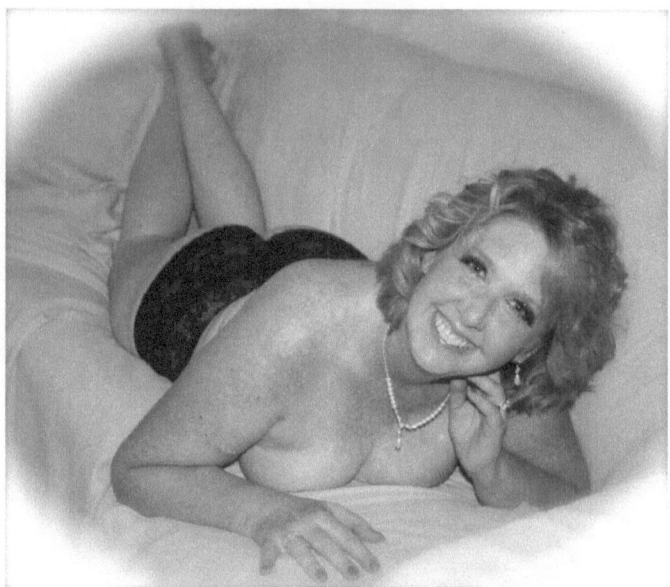

I wanted you to see that I do feel sexy. Most of the time, I forget that this procedure has even been done. I guess I mean I feel this way when I'm doing my daily business. It is not something I am conscious of.

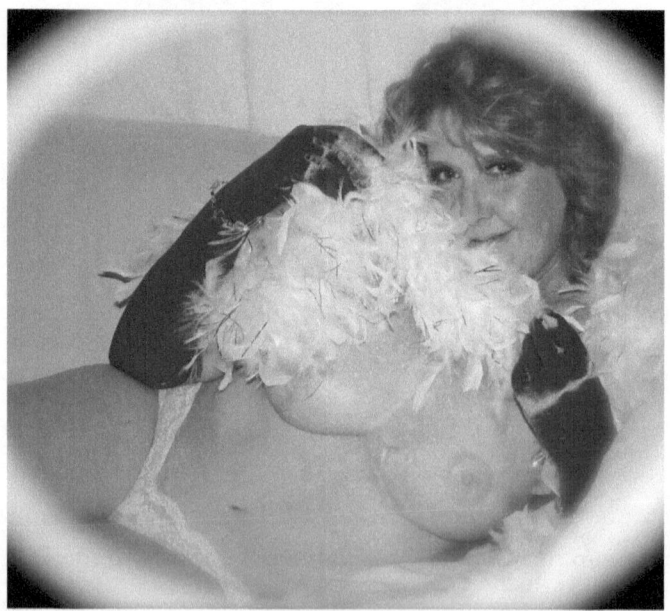

Like I said, *you can still feel sexy after this. It doesn't have to ruin your life.* You can be sexy all you want!

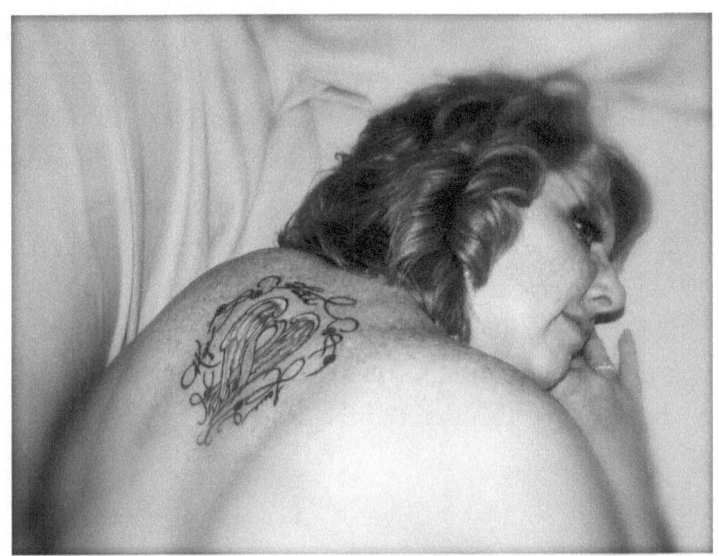

My tattoo and my guardian angel—always with me!

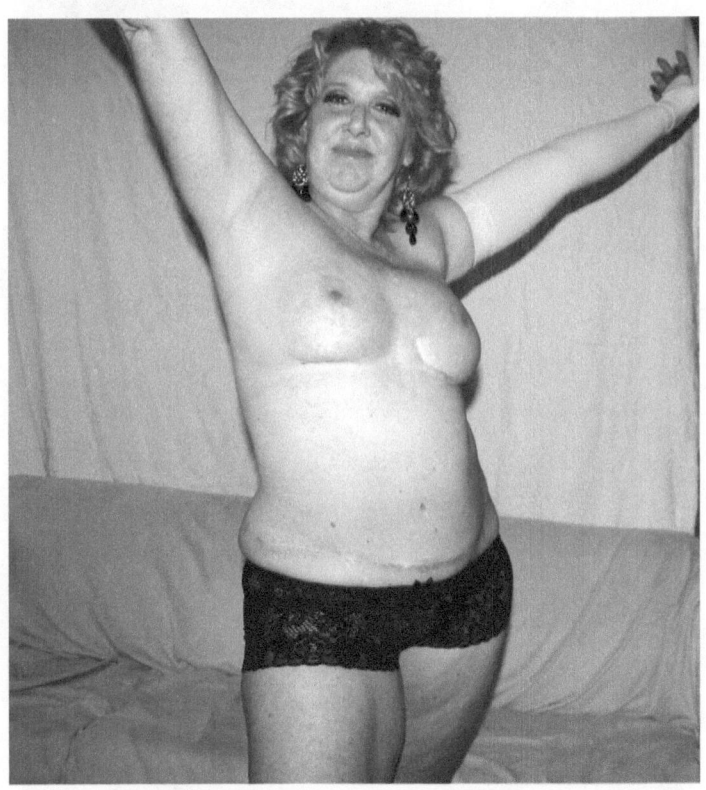

Let's celebrate! I am cancer-free! And this is me!

These next photos I owe to Rebecca Sharp with Sharp Images. She kindly donated her time to take these photos for me. They were taken In August 2013. I would urge *anyone* who wants a good photographer to look her up! She does some wonderful Boudoir photos and makes you feel right at home. I thank her so much for her hard work! *These are the most recent photos.* I want you to understand when you are looking at these that she made *every* effort to *not glamorize me*! We were trying to make sure that you got to see *exactly* what I looked like. It was a chore for her. Her job is to glamorize, and she had to try hard *not* to! So here we go. Thanks, Rebecca. Look her up!

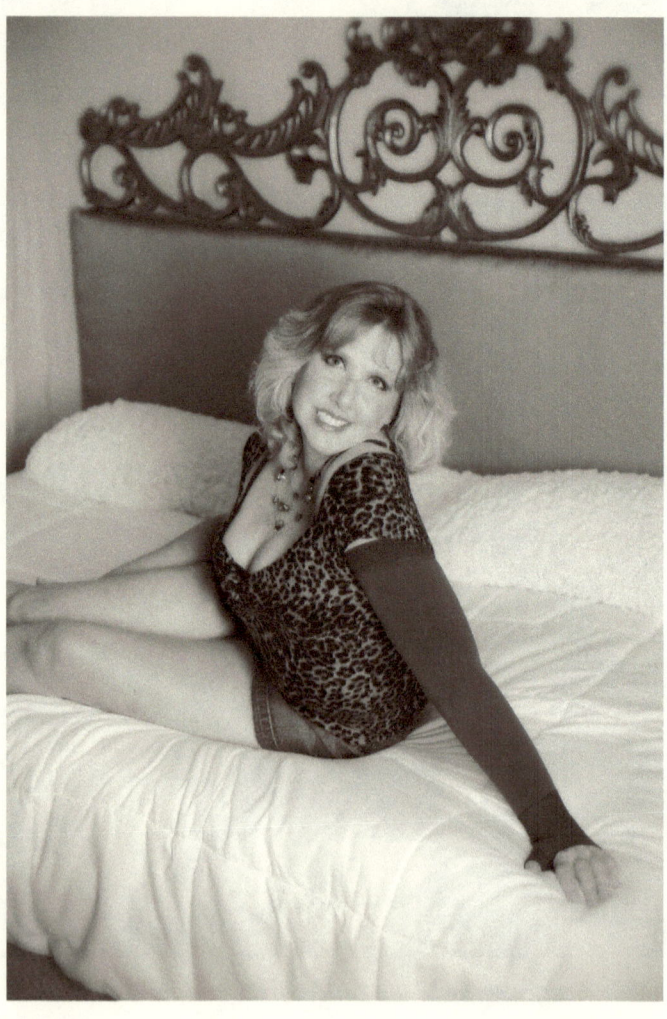

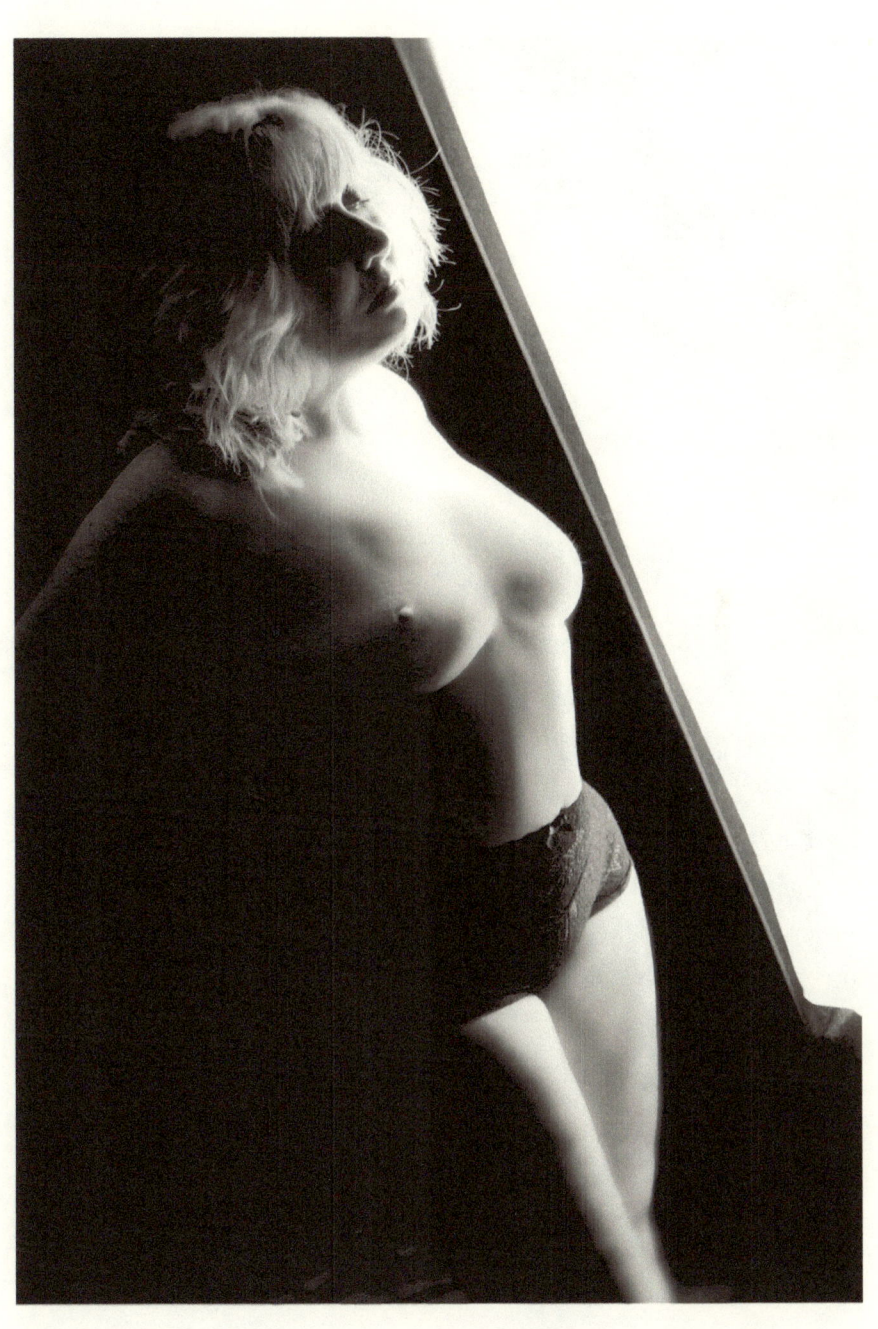

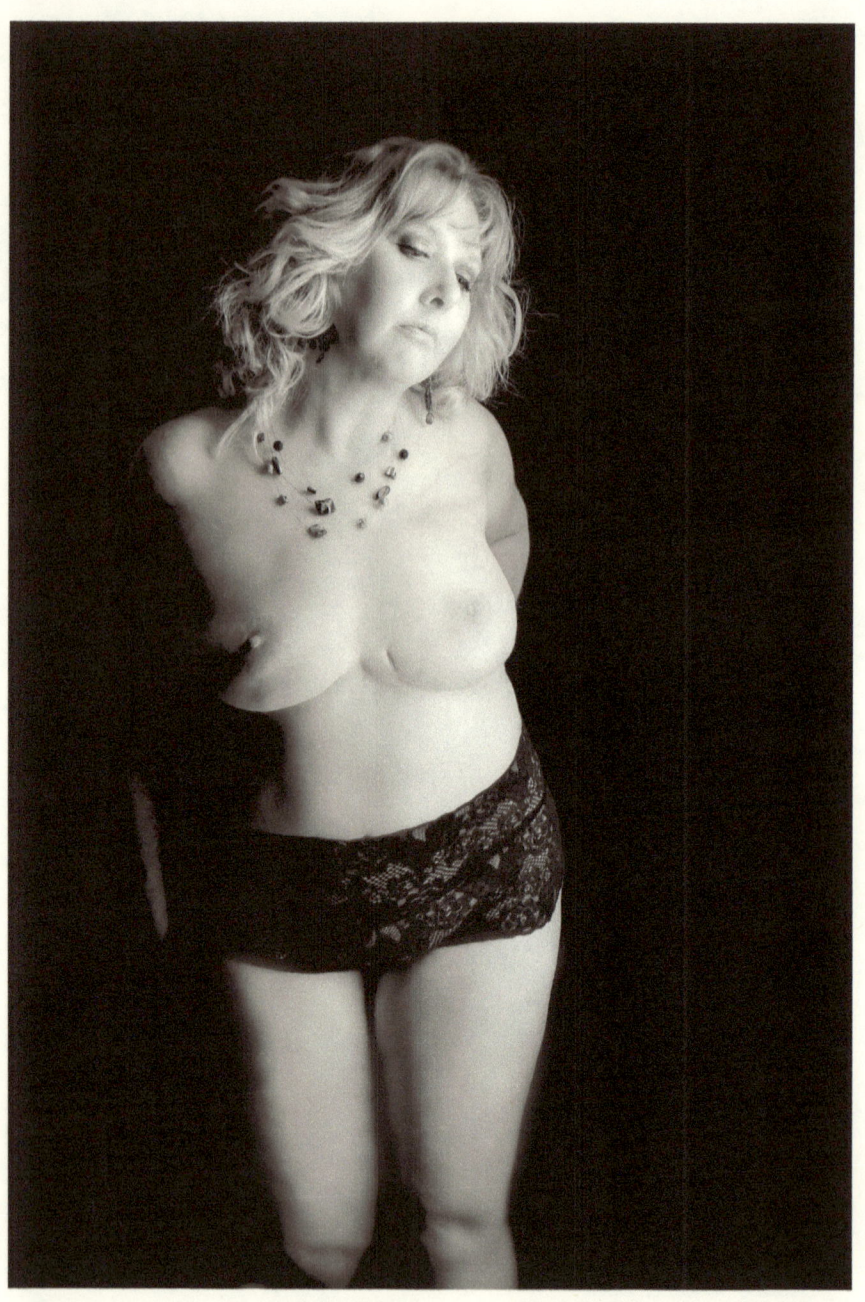

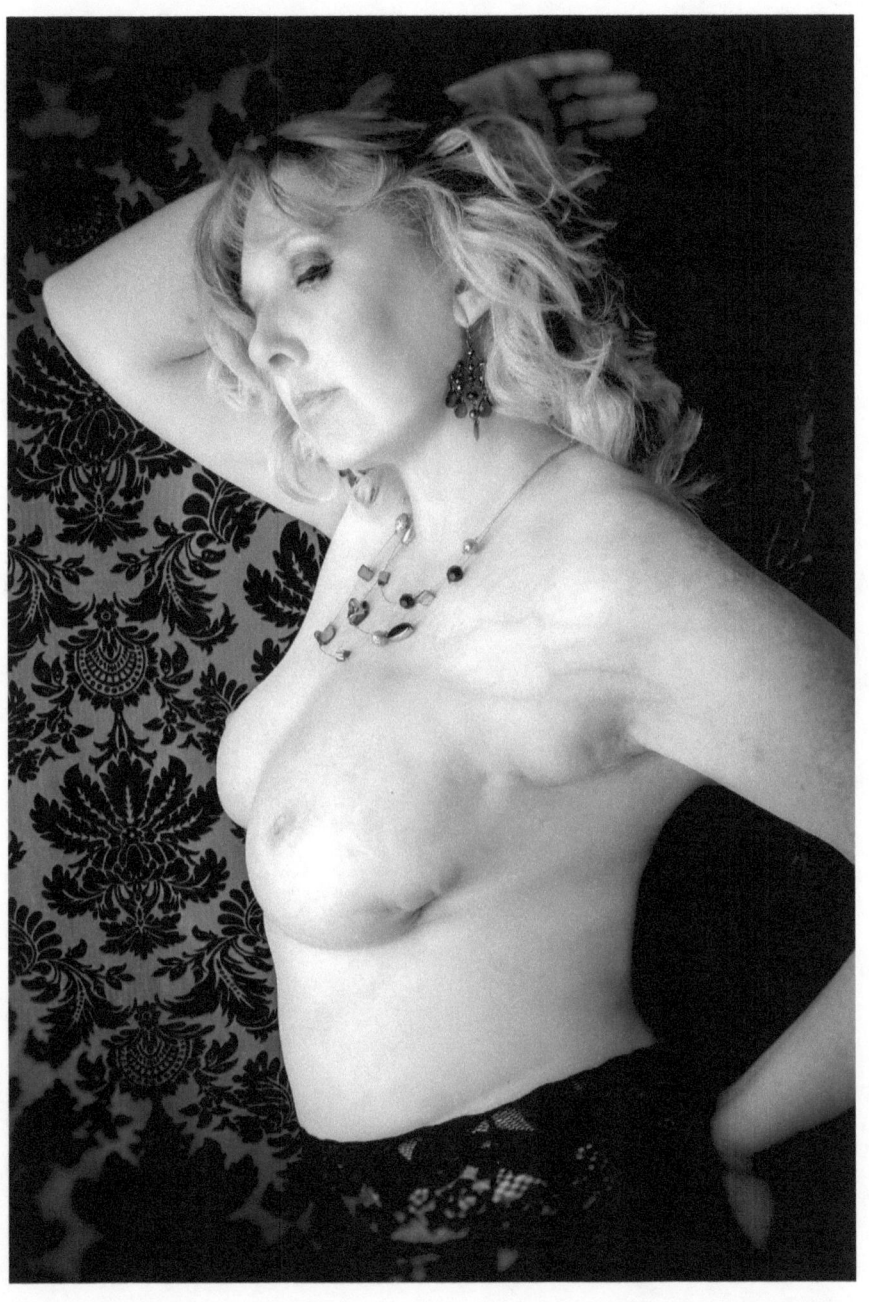

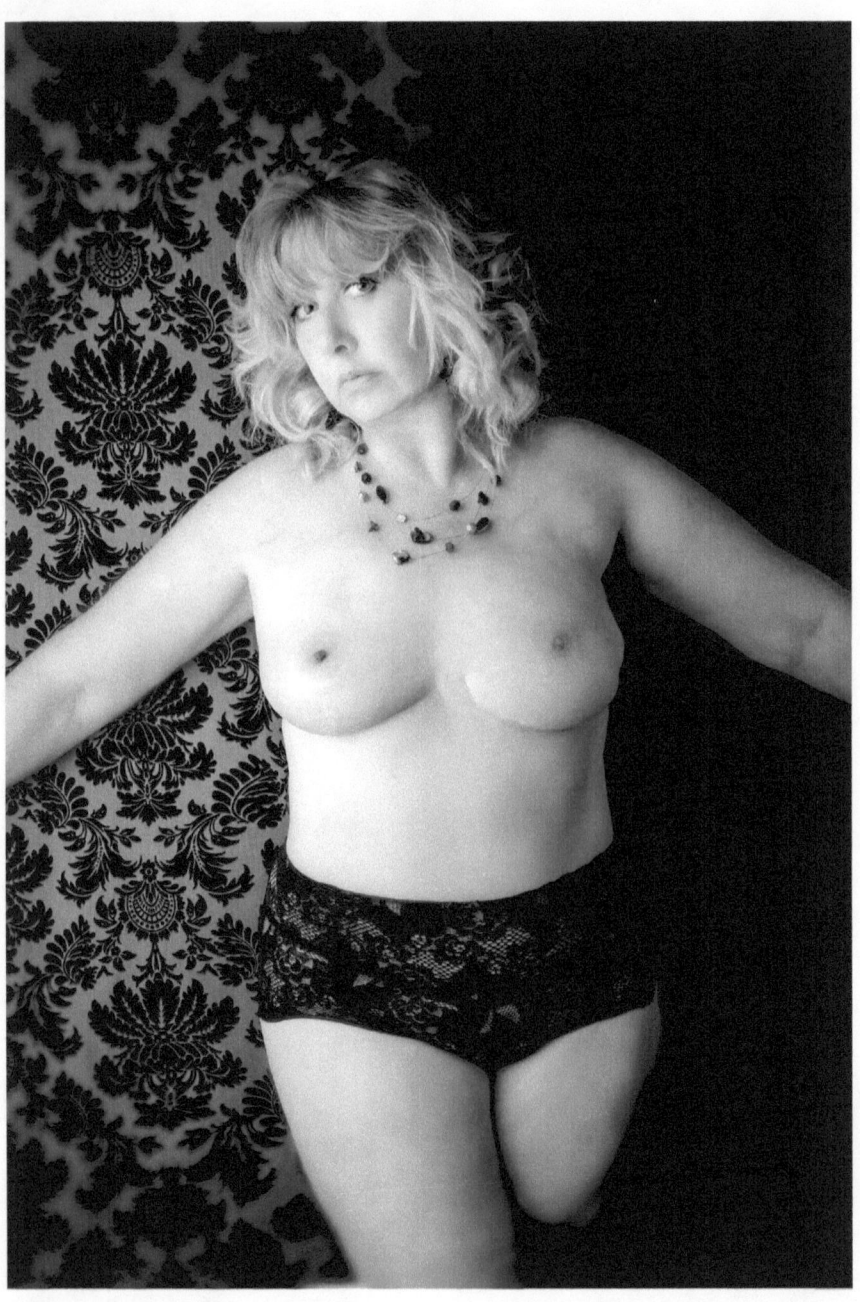

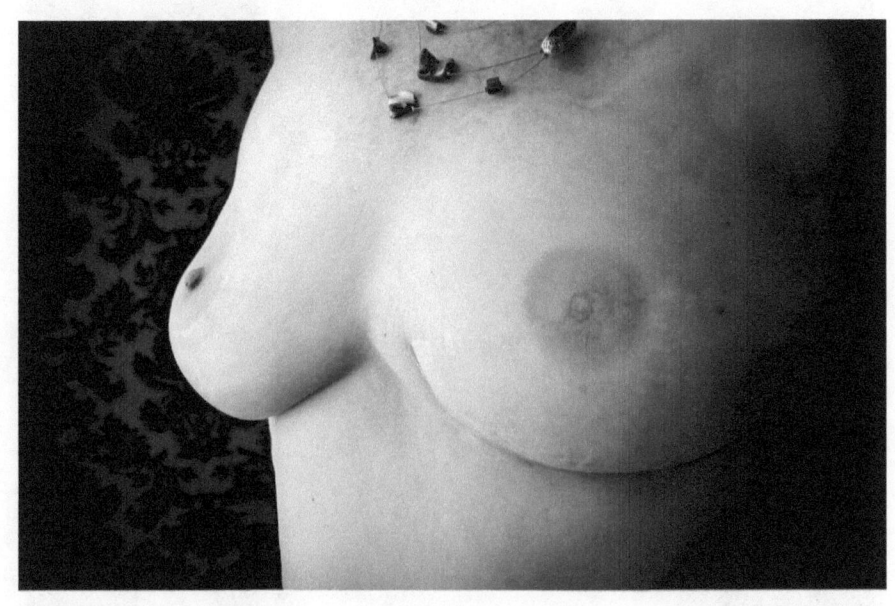

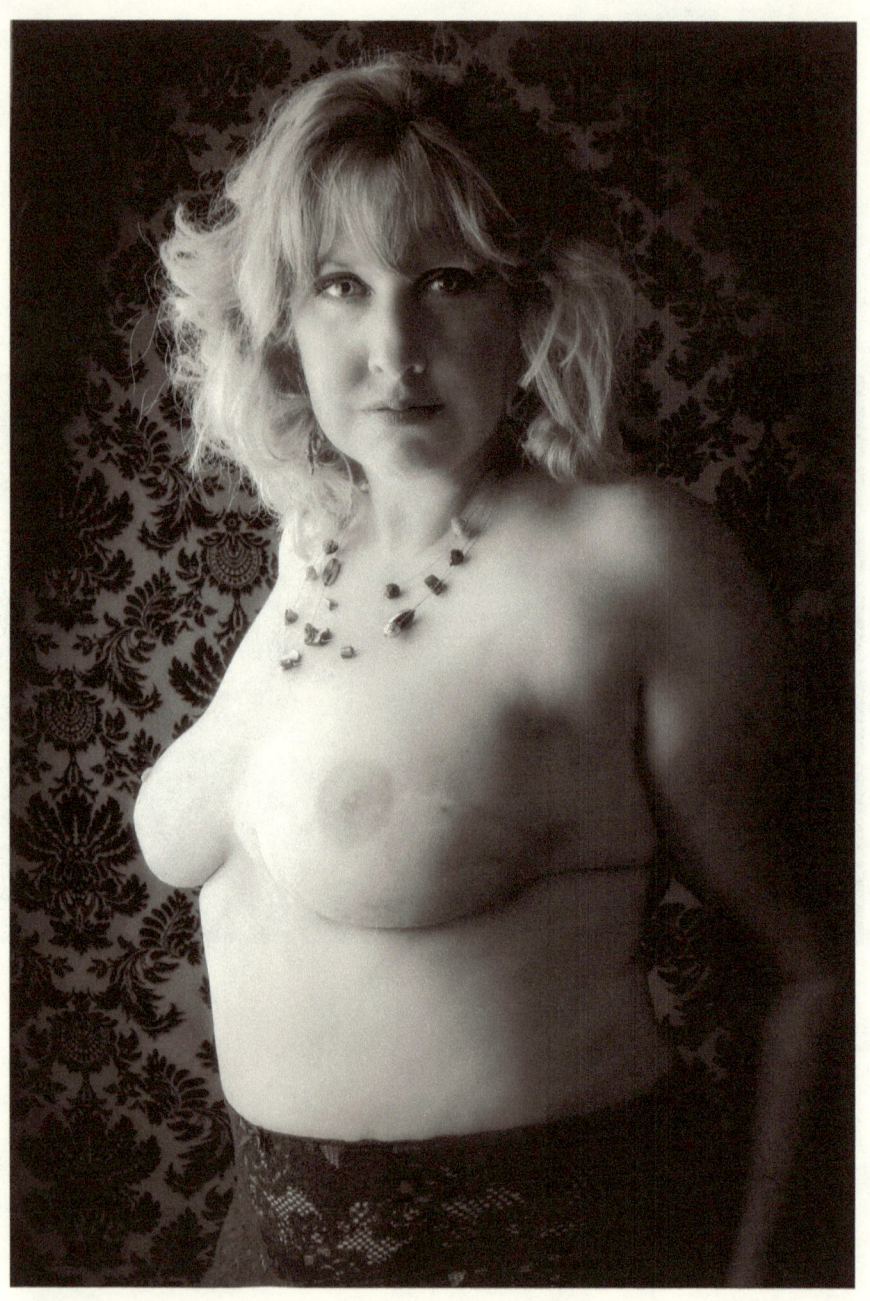

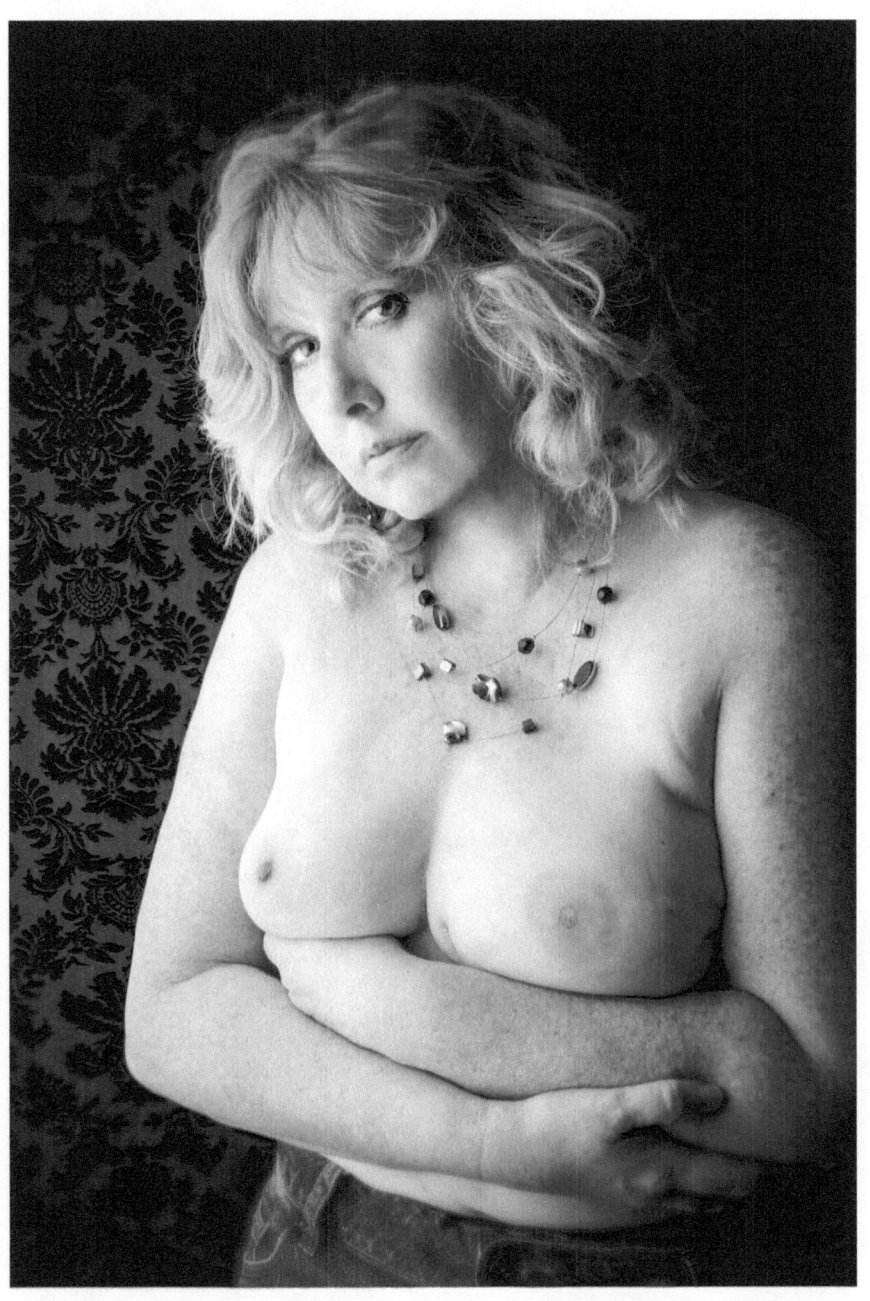

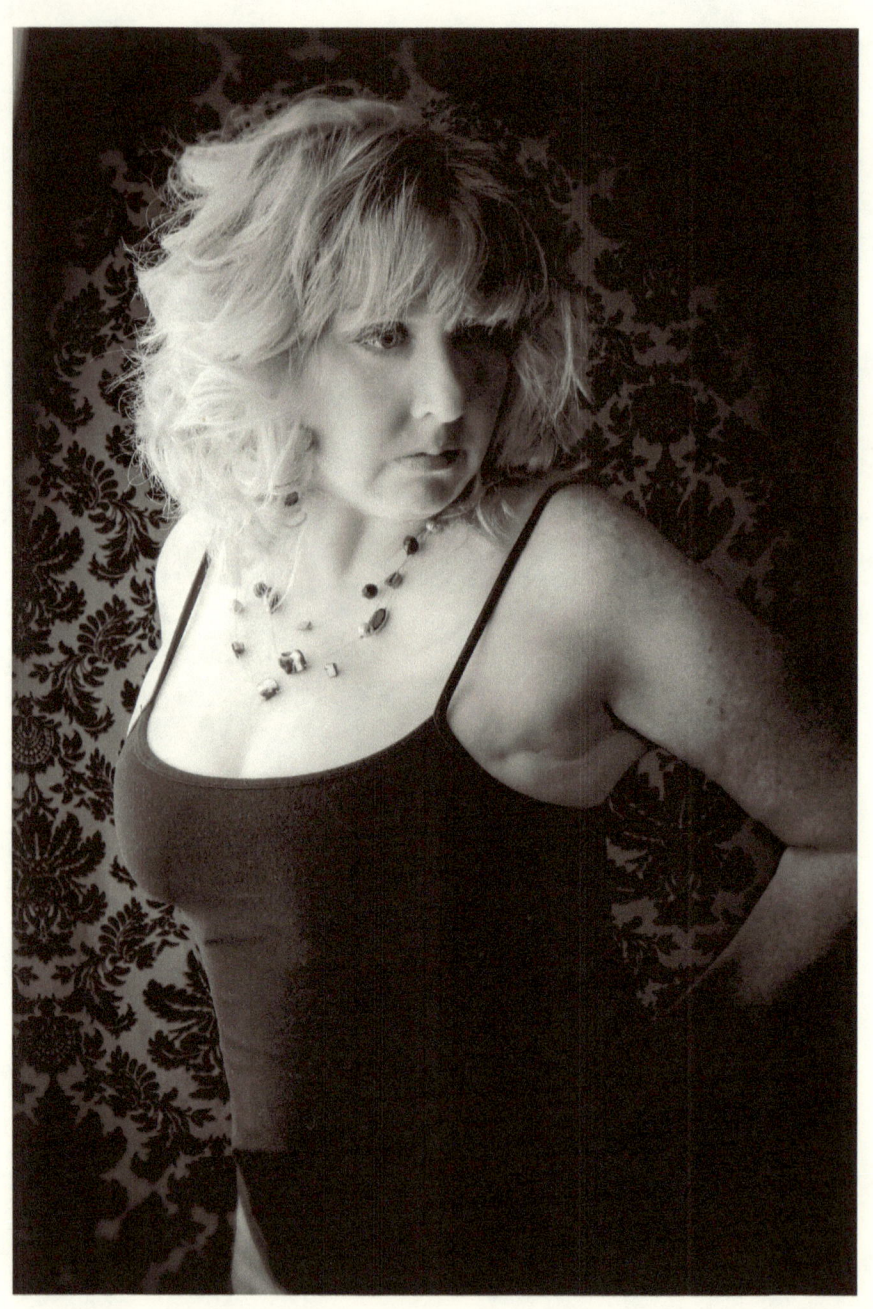

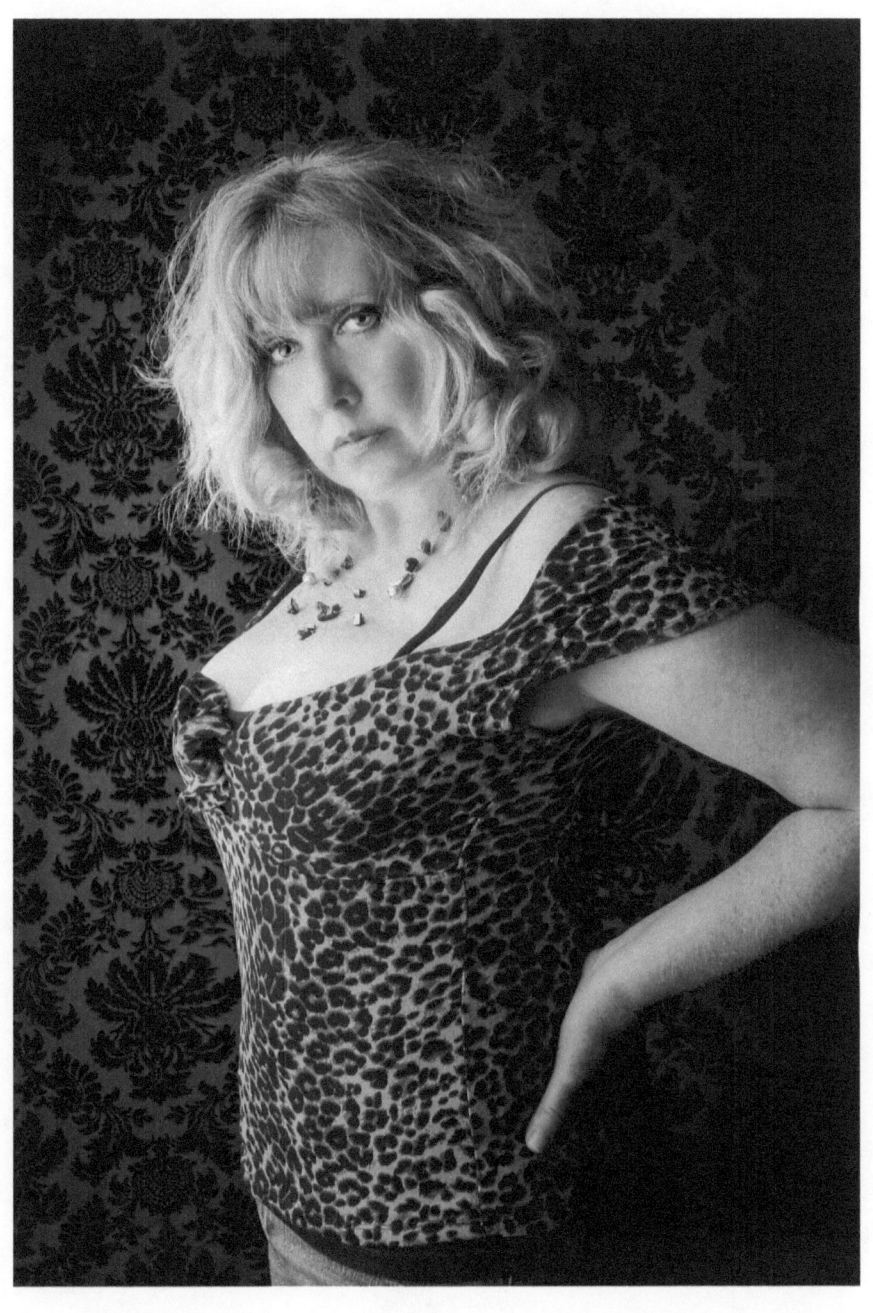

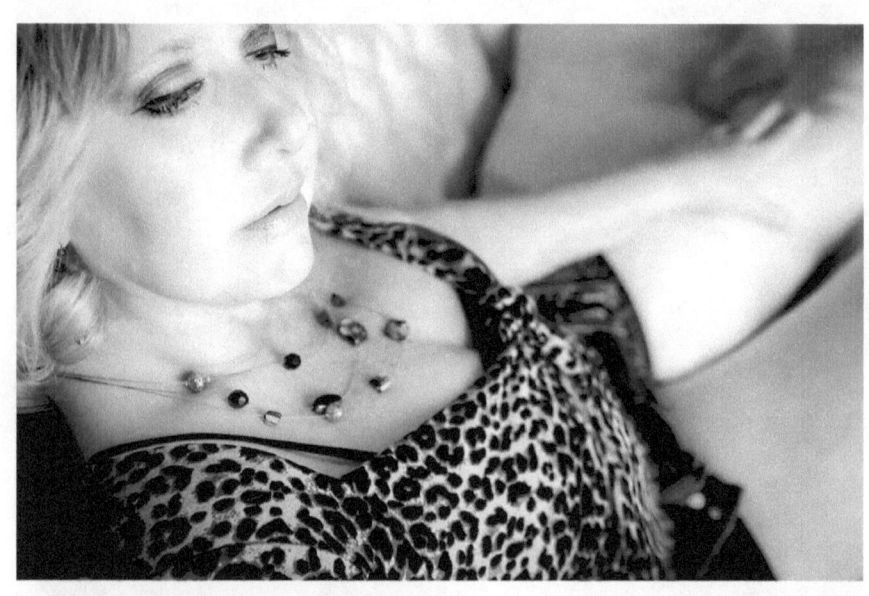
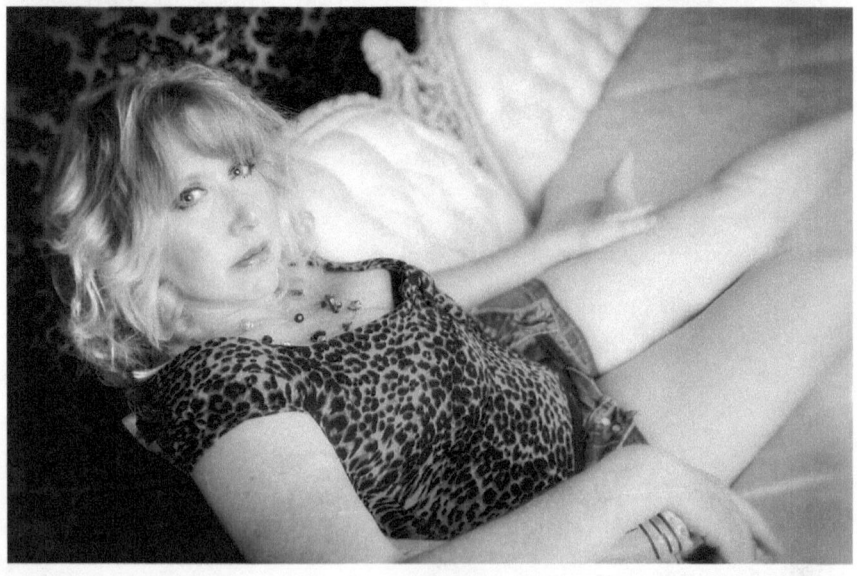

Chapter 5

"Chemo Information"

Well, you've seen what has happened with the whole mastectomy and reconstruction. Now, I specifically chose the mastectomy with the hope and implication that I would *not* need chemotherapy or radiation therapy. It was implied all along that once the mastectomy was done, I was home free, so to speak.

I never even thought about going back to the oncologist after my mastectomy. I didn't hear from them, and no one mentioned that I should visit him.

So I la-di-da wandered into my surgeon's office for a follow-up visit six weeks or so after the mastectomy, at which time we discussed everything, when suddenly she said, "So what did the oncologist have to say about your pathology report?" I whipped my head around like in *The Exorcist*! *What?* "I'm sorry? Oncologist?" She then seemed confused by my confusion. (This is why I say to *ask lots of questions*.) *Well, it seems that I was to see the oncologist!* Duh! I should have known this, huh? *No!*

Honestly, there is so much going on between doctors that one doctor might have thought the other doctor told me to go. I don't know, but this was a complete shock and startled me! She said I should have seen him a few weeks after the surgery. *Crap!*

So I made the appointment, still thinking even after my conversation with my surgeon that it still was unlikely that chemo would be needed. At this point, we were getting close to Christmas time. I believe my appointment was on December 20.

It seemed that the pathology report after the removal of the mass showed that the type of cancer and the size and the depth—well, it would make the chances of my cancer recurring to under 3 percent if I did the chemotherapy. Without it, honestly, I can't remember the percentage, but it was *much* higher than 3 percent. It was a no-brainer. I had to do it.

I was scared. Of course, one of the first questions I asked was "Will I lose my hair?" He said, "Well, unfortunately, this drug *does* cause most people to lose their hair. I have seen very few that haven't, but most people do. But *it's just hair. It will grow back.*" He is a kind, soft-spoken man. And in the overall scheme of things, he is right. It *is* just hair. The option at this point in my life was to give up my hair to save my life. Well, OK; guess that's a good trade-off.

On a side note, now would be a good time for you to go to whatever organization you can to get fitted for a wig while you still have your hair. They can get you one that looks identical to what you have, but I chose to get one totally different. I got a cute redheaded wig. Also, *get hats, scarves,* and *turbans.* Ask your doctor for a list of locations for such. If they don't know, contact the American Cancer Society. They will be able to provide you with the closest location.

Everyone is different in how they handle the loss of their hair. It is a personal thing. It really didn't bother me. I have a *massive amount* of hair, so it saved me about thirty minutes of getting ready! Many times my dad would ask me, "You about ready to go?" In which I would reply, "Yep, just gotta do my hair!" He had to think about it for a minute or two on the first few times I said it, but then it was just a joke. First off, you only have to use about a drop of shampoo, and then, *no styling.* Slip on a hat, and that's it! *I loved it!* And think of all the money you'll save on hair supplies!

So let's go! I would start my first treatment right after the first of the year. I still had questions. "What exactly *is* chemo?" "How does it work?" "What will you do?" etc.

He showed me around and introduced me to the nurses. (It's very important to know these people! You want to get on their good side. *Bring treats!*) He showed me the rooms and the chairs. But it still wasn't enough.

Let me tell you what happens—what my experience was. Now remember that chemotherapy is very different for every person. Same as cancer. No two people have the same exact reaction or handle it the same way. So just because I had things happen to me a certain way, that doesn't mean that it will happen to you like this. It only gives you an *idea* of what *can* happen.

They set me up for my appointment and said I could count on being there for about four hours and they'd see me then! *What?*

OK then. They also prescribe *massive* doses of steroids before the treatment, during the treatment, and right after the treatment. This has been known to help with the nausea from the treatment. I must say it did seem to help.

My steroid was in a pill form; I was to take a dose the day before, the day of, and then the day after. *Now,* there *are* side effects from the steroids that you *should* read very carefully on the little side-effect sheet that comes with your medication.

The first day I took the medicine, I was feeling quite peppy. I was a bit nervous about going for the treatment the next day, but at this point, what could be so bad, right? But just the word *chemo* is scary, right?

Well, the next day came. I showed up with two bags full of stuff to do. They were cracking up at me. Like I was moving in! They will tell you to bring a pillow if you want for comfort and anything you want to keep yourself occupied with. Well, I get bored easy, so I had my computer and plenty of stuff to work on! (You really don't need to bring two suitcases full of stuff; it was a bit over-the-top!)

They took me into a room; there were several other people there. It was a bit intimidating, but that is how it is in some cancer-treatment centers. They do have some private rooms, but there is a chance you will go into a "community cancer room." In the end, I didn't mind. I had people to talk to. Their caregivers were there, waiting with them. *I highly recommend that you always have someone with you.* You never know what your reaction might be or how you might feel.

I got all situated in my chair, and they said they would be right back to get started. I took a scan of the other patients. They all seemed to be doing fine. They were reading, taking naps, etc. Most of them were just with an IV in their arms; a few had ports. For those of you that don't know what a *port* is, it is a semipermanent IV that is generally placed in the chest area. It has a cap on it, and if you are having long-term treatments, it makes it easier on you and them to apply the drugs. The cap keeps it clean, and it just pops off when they need it. If they have to do numerous treatments, there is a chance that your veins will collapse. This is *not* a horrible thing; it is just another way to treat you. It might be a little inconvenient, but not a horrible thing. When you are all done with your treatment, the port comes out. I *did not* have to have a port. I managed to just have the IV treatment every time. I was lucky; I only had to have four treatments, one every three weeks.

With the scan of the other patients, it didn't seem to be so bad.

The nurse came back and said, "OK, we'll get started."

"OK. *How do we do that?*"

She said, "I'll just get the IV started, then we just change out the bags. You have three to go through. Once you go through the three bags, you are done. We like to start with the steroid then the other two cancer drugs. We will start them all with a slow drip, and if you are handling them OK, then we will speed them up a little bit. If you have any reaction, feel poorly—anything at all, we stop the drug *immediately*, make sure you are OK, then we start again until we finish." Then she handed me a bell; yes, a bell. "If you feel *anything at all*, you *must* ring the bell, and we will come right away."

I was like OK, but I had no idea what I *might feel*. (At one of my treatments, I did have some back pain. I really thought and still think that I needed to reposition in the chair, but the nurse happened to be in there, she said that it could have been a reaction. So they stopped the treatment and waited, and then we started again. It took *forever*. But that is what they mean. I still wouldn't have rung the bell because I have back pain anyway. They might be more specific about what you might feel, but they mostly are concerned with headache, nausea, etc.)

OK. It seemed reasonable. An IV—like I hadn't had a million of those started in my lifetime! She got it in and started the session. I felt *nothing*—absolutely *nothing*. I didn't feel sick. I didn't feel like I was on fire. I didn't feel like *anything*. It was perfectly fine. *I went out to eat afterward.*

Now the next day, I felt like I had drunk ten five-hour energy drinks. I hopped out of bed and proceeded to clean the *whole house*! I was like the Energizer Bunny. I had *so* much energy I didn't know what to do! It was the steroid.

Now, I *did* have a little problem. They say it was *not* related to the chemo or the steroid, but that very day after my cleaning spree, I was taking a shower and promptly passed out cold. I mean, *I passed out*. I had just enough time to pound on the wall and call out to my mom and to slide down into the tub. Thank goodness! But then I was out.

(I have weird things that happen to me though.)

I didn't feel well after that that day. But the next day, I was fine. I was fine until day *seven*. Day *seven* was my day to start feeling bad. It wasn't horrible, but I felt like I had the flu. My stomach cramped, and I ached a bit, and I was worn out. I basically stayed in bed for the *next* four to six days. Usually, by the seventh day, I was magically better again. Now, there will come a time that you have a huge drop in your white blood cells, making you extremely vulnerable to *anything*. It was usually about the time I started to feel better. That window lasts about seven days. Then it's time to go back for another treatment. You can still go out during that time, but you *must* be careful. I had masks, and I had antibacterial wipes. I wiped down tables at restaurants and their menus, sometimes the utensils. I was particularly conscious of doors and bathrooms. Really, anything that others touched. I wasn't afraid to keep an antibacterial wipe out to open and close doors. *It is your life!*

And yes, I did lose my hair. It only took about two weeks after the first treatment. I kept waiting and waiting, tugging on my hair every day. I had already cut it fairly short. When suddenly, I pulled and got a handful of hair then another and another and another. It was kind of fun pulling it out. I have a *lot of hair*! *I mean—a lot!* I wondered how long it would take for it all to come out. My nephew (Christopher Conway), *God bless him*, he was a super strong buddy for me. Anyway, he was lying in my room with me, keeping me company, and we were both pulling out pieces of my hair. He was so worried about me losing my hair. I wasn't so worried about it. I knew it was going to happen, and I was prepared. Mentally, I was prepared. The more I pulled the pieces out, the more that seemed to fall all around me. *Eeeeewwwwwww! If* I let this go on, I was going to wake up coughing out a fur ball! So I told Chris, "*I must shave this off!*" He said, "*No, Aunt Dana!* Maybe it won't all fall out!" I told him calmly it was OK. That yes, it was time. That it would be OK. I went into the bathroom, and guess what? There were no signs of a shaver. I was certain we had one. All I had was my little personal shaver. *Oh well.* Had to make do with what I got. So I started. Zip-a-dee-doo-da, zip-a-dee-ya! It was kind of cool. I felt like it was empowering in a little bit of a way; like the chemo wasn't in control of this part, but I *was*. So there I was shaving, but as I said, I have a *lot of hair*; it is *very* thick. My dad came in and saw what I was doing. He was totally shocked. I could see the sadness in his eyes. He asked if he could do the back of my hair for me. I told him yes; it would be awesome since I couldn't see the back of my head! Together, we shaved it off. I didn't mind it. It was done. Now my head was *cold*. Here is the need for the *caps*. I never knew how important having the right kind of one would be. So to all you people that will lose your hair, *your head will get cold*, and you need to find hats and nightcaps. Reach out to your local cancer societies, accept their help, and don't be afraid to take different ones. Because when you sleep at night, *your head will get cold*!

Well, unfortunately, your hair may not be the only thing that you lose while going through chemotherapy. I wasn't aware of this fun thing... loss of taste. No wonder people lose weight and don't want to eat when they are going through this! I wasn't really prepared for this, but it happened, and what a weird, weird thing! I thank God for letting me still be able to taste chocolate! I have no idea how that happened. It's like the one thing I would wish for, (if I COULD have,) to be able to taste. That, AND I could taste REALLY, REALLY spicy salsa. But, sometimes I would pay for that. It didn't always set well with my stomach. It's a really hard thing to explain, I mean you know that when you are putting mashed potatoes and gravy in your mouth that it should taste like mashed potatoes and gravy, but instead, it tastes like... well, nothing, not even water tastes right.

This too, returns to normal after your treatment ends. Some people don't even have to face this. But, just in case, be prepared for it, or at least ask your doctor if it is a side effect of your treatment. It is quite a shock if you aren't prepared for it. When your taste buds start returning to normal it's shocking as well. You'll be eating, and not even thinking about it, when suddenly you'll realize that "HEY! I can taste this!"

I found that making sure you have the nutrition shakes on hand is very helpful. Sometimes you just don't feel like eating, especially when you know you are going to be disappointed. But YOU HAVE TO STAY NOURISHED. So, this is one thing you MUST do to fight this fight! Even though you might not enjoy eating or drinking the shakes, just try to as much as you can. Your body needs as much help to stay strong as you can give it.

Also, sometimes, if you keep trying different foods, you might just find something that you CAN taste, and then you can at least have that to look forward to! And, I, of course, GAINED weight during chemo...I mean WHO gains weight during chemo? I did. My Oncologist was always thrilled. I was not so much, and would not share in the celebration!

My dad would bring me a chocolate shake, or some chocolate candy. It was always very sweet of him to think of me and it was his way of helping me try to eat.

What an interesting thing this chemo is, huh? It kills everything. We feel like crap. We have hope for success. We finish it. Then hope everything goes back to normal. What would we do without it? Many, many people would be dead. We must be grateful for this treatment, it is what saves lives.

Following are pictures of my shaven head!

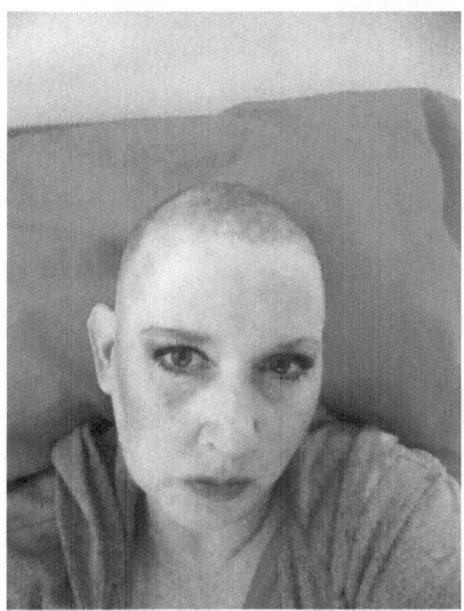

Taken January 2011.

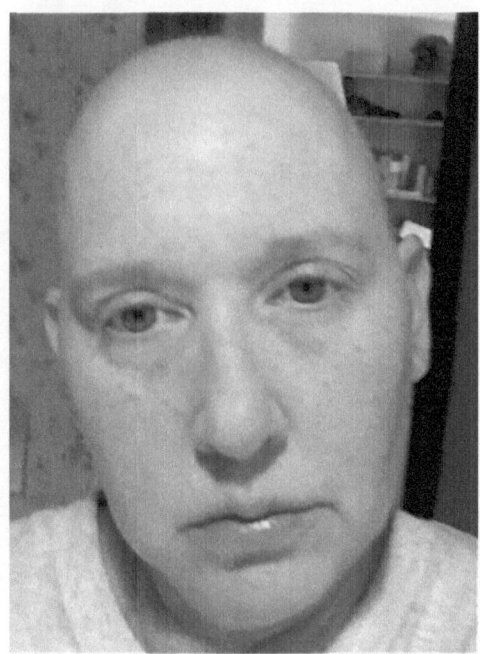

Taken during my last chemo treatment, March 2011.

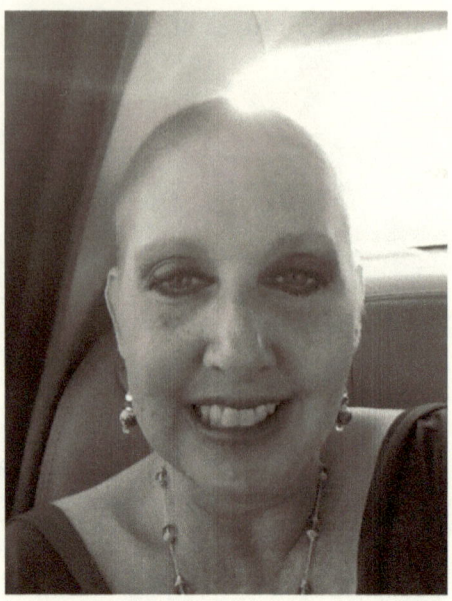

My last chemo treatment was in March. This was taken
in June, so as you can see, I have some hair growth.
By Christmas, I had a complete head of hair.

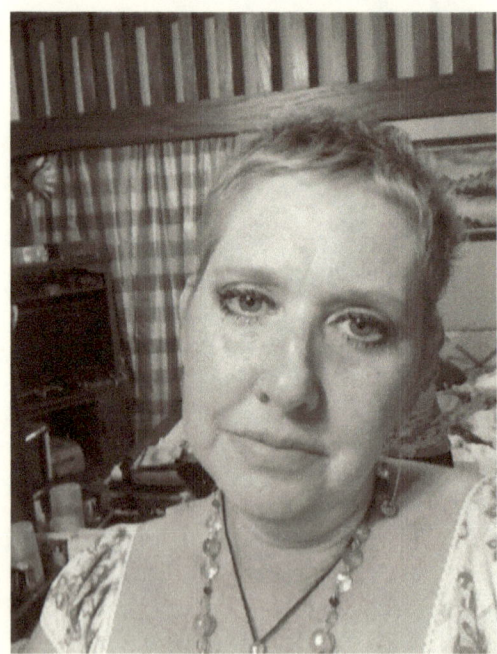

July 2011

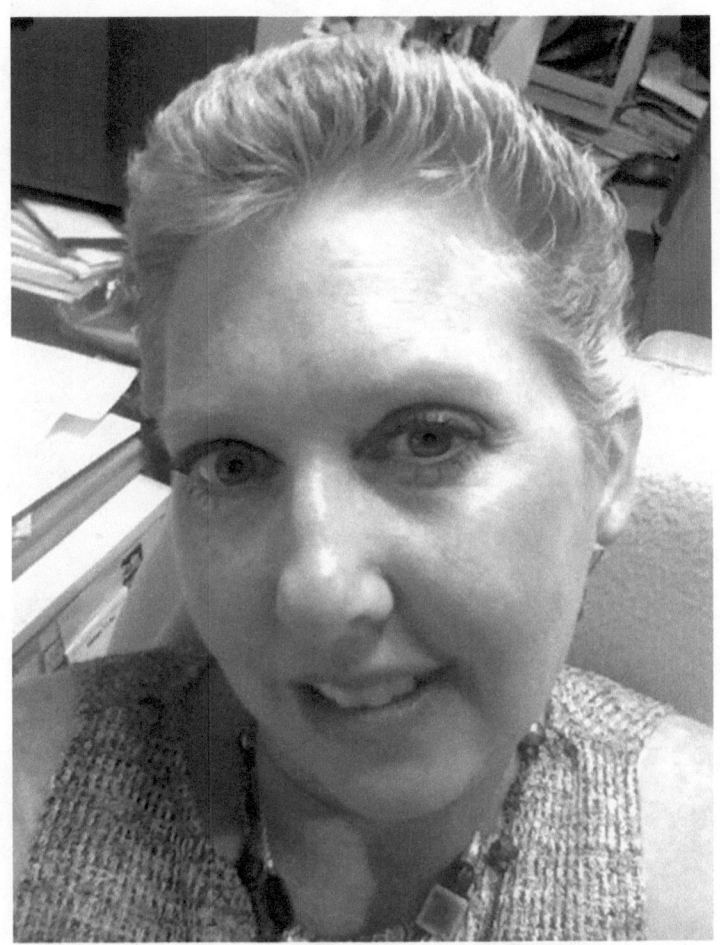

July 2011

October 2011 with my beautiful niece.

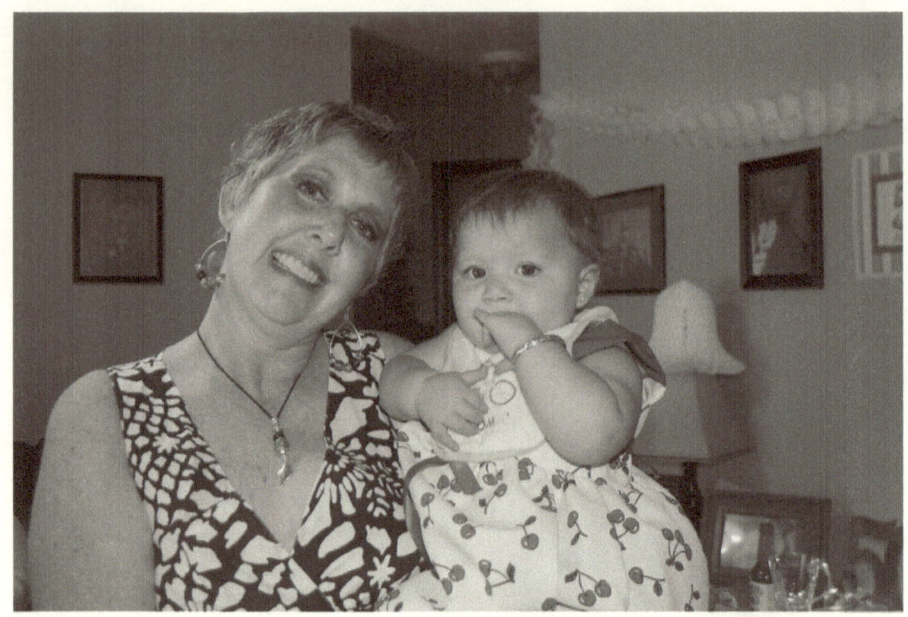

Celestra

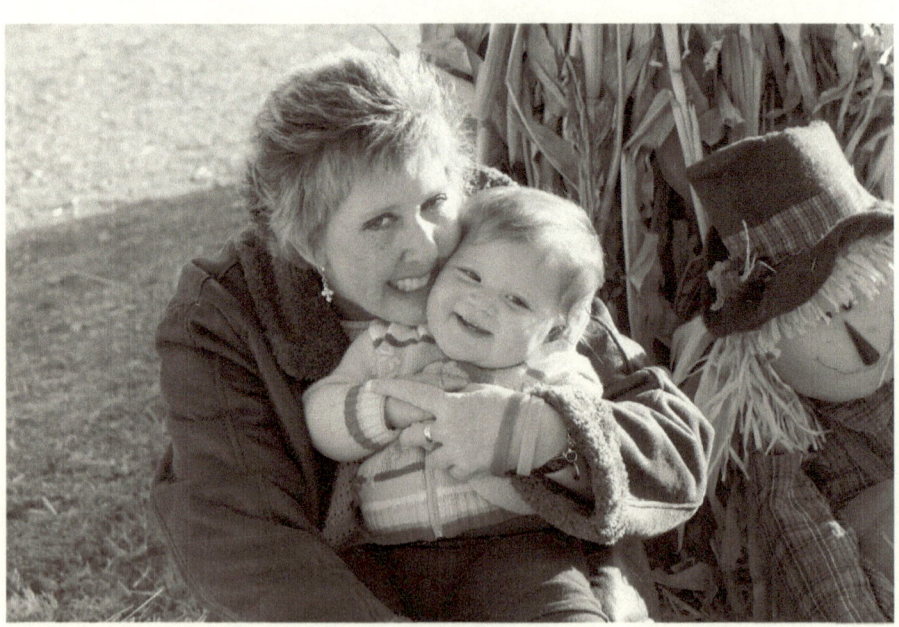

Conway!

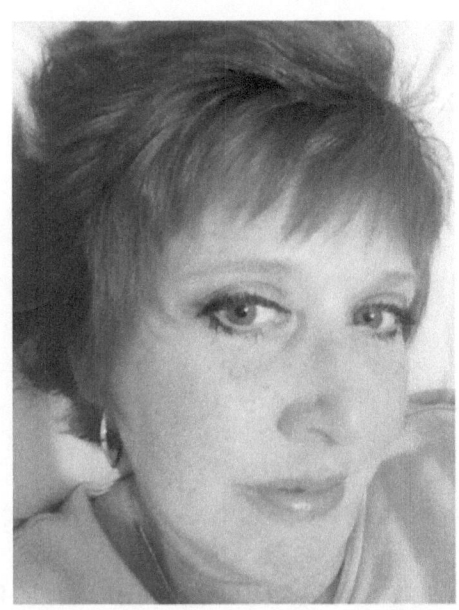

December 2011
This gives you some idea of how long it might take to get your hair back.

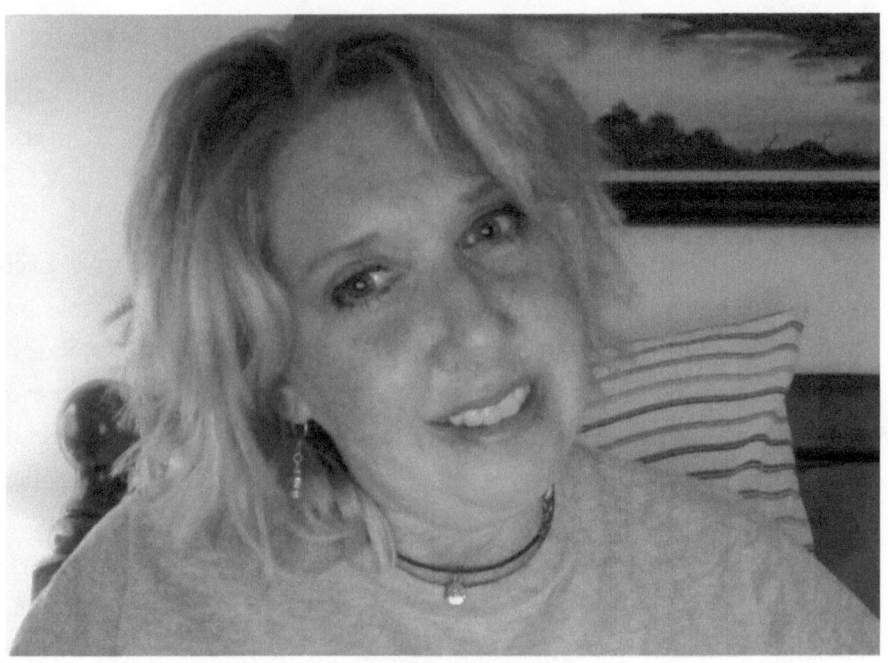

November 2012
More than I started with!

Chapter 6

"My Cancer Story"

applaud you for taking time to do research and to read my stories. I hope that it helps you some. Everyone has their cancer story. It is not my intention to take away from your battle. I do want you to know that you aren't alone and that there is *hope* to make it through this. I would like to share a little bit about my history and how I found my cancer.

It was May of 2010. I was in the hospital, just coming out of back surgery. My now ex-husband of twenty-two years was there in the room with me, as well as my mom and dad and son.

My ex and I had been having problems for a while, but it was not ever feasible for me to leave the situation. Divorce was not acceptable on his part. My son had just finished his junior year in high school and was about to turn seventeen. That day changed my life forever. It was a horrible experience. My ex accused me of having an affair. He waited until all my family had left the hospital, and *then* he let me have it. He had my phone in his hand and awoke me by throwing it at my back. I'd rather not go into all the details, as it was rather nasty. Long story short, this night would be the last night for us. My parents moved me, as well as my son, in with them after I got out of the hospital. I then had some complications with the surgery and a blood clot in my left leg. It took weeks to heal.

I had worked at my office-manager position for twenty-one years. I returned to work and was getting back into a routine and trying to get used to the idea of getting divorced. I found that I could be strong. I could deal with this. I *am* strong.

I was continuing with a plan. The divorce was not a pleasant one. I don't know many that are. I was coping. My son was coping. We were trying to move on. On September 28, 2010, I was taking my dogs outside. It was a little cold, so I had my hands crossed over my chest when—*Huh? What is that!* On my left breast, close to the nipple, I felt a lump. I immediately felt it again, hoping the neighbors weren't watching. Yep, there was something there. I tried to console myself by saying, "I just had a mammogram done in July, and it was *all clear!*" But something deep inside me knew that this was not normal and it was something to be concerned about.

I lost my aunt Ruby to breast cancer. She was my mom's eldest sister. When she found the lump and before she had her mastectomy, she insisted that we *felt* it. Thank you, *Aunt Ruby*. I have had people ask me, what does it feel like? I wish I could have them feel it. All I can say is that it doesn't feel like a fibrocystic anything. It is completely different. Mine was near the nipple, so I *knew* that wasn't right. It had never been there before. It was *hard*, and it did not move. It was definitely different from any other lump I'd ever felt. When they say you should do self breast exams, this is why—because you become familiar with your body, and when something is out of place, *you know it*. I knew it.

This was a Saturday when I found it. I went inside and told my mom about it. She felt it, and the look on her face told me that my reaction was correct. She said it didn't feel normal to her. We decided to wait until the next day and see how it felt then. Sunday came, and there was no difference. I was then to call my doctor on Monday to let her know what I found.

The call was made, and she was equally concerned.

I would have another mammogram. They were concerned. You can see it in everyone's eyes when there is that possibility. I already knew. But they have to have proof. So they would schedule a biopsy. (See biopsy what the heck?) I found out on my daddy's birthday, October 7, 2010, that yes, it was cancer.

The next thing we did was see the surgeon on that following Monday. I have had the pleasure of doing business with Dr. Long on other occasions. Now, she would be in charge of guiding me through making decisions about breast cancer.

So many decisions. So many things to think about. I had already premeditated mastectomy. But they were considering just a lumpectomy, followed by a lot of chemo and radiation. Again, gathering information about what your particular cancer is and what treatment choices you have is a daunting task. It pays to do your research. Look online; look at the reliable sources through the American Cancer Society and so forth. Also, *don't* always take what you read on the Internet as the gospel truth. Use it as a tool to get more information from your doctors. The more information you have, the more questions you can ask and the better decision you can make for yourself.

After many appointments with the oncologist and the radiologist and more tests, including an MRI (which is *the best form of detection of breast cancer*, by the way), they found several other areas of suspicion. With that, I decided on the mastectomy of my left breast with reconstruction of the right breast. Then came all the discussion about reconstruction. The plastic surgeon, another doctor I had the pleasure of doing prior business with (and no, it was not cosmetic!), would give me several options as well. My final decision was to go with the TRAM procedure. (See the pics of recovery.) So all those decisions were made.

I had a discussion with my employer about my cancer and the treatment options and what would be coming my way. Due to a confidentiality clause, I am not permitted to discuss anything further than this.

I can say that I am unemployed. I have been unemployed since October 2010.

I was then facing a divorce, cancer, and no income.

I must tell you that really, at that moment and time, the only thing that mattered was fighting for my life. I had to put all my positive energy into fighting this thing! I was going to make it. I never doubted that I could survive this. It would be OK. I don't want you to think that it was ever a breeze; it wasn't. But all of this has given me an ability to have *faith*.

I must share one final story with you that happened when I went to the hospital for my surgery.

I hope that you can have an open mind and that this will touch your heart in some way.

I had just come up to my room from my surgery—the mastectomy and the reconstruction all at the same time. The surgery was approximately six hours long. Some of this I am repeating from my mother because I don't remember. She states that she walked into the room, and the nurses were slapping me and yelling at me, trying to get me to breathe. My mom said to them, "What is going on in here!" They explained that I was not breathing properly and that if I didn't improve *quickly*, I would need to be intubated.

My mom asked if she could try to get me awake enough to breathe for them. They said, "Sure, try!" So (I remember this well) she said to me, "Dana, I know you think you are breathing, but you are not. You need to wake up, and you need to take a deep breath for me." I heard her barely. I was thinking in my head, *I am breathing, or else I'd be dead! But* I took a breath, and they had a little party. I did it again, and everyone was happy. However, this whole waking-me-up-and-making-me-breathe continued on and on with different people taking turns—my mom, Betty Conway; my cousin Denise McConnell; my sister-in-law Kristie Conway; my nephew Dallas Conway; my dad, Jerry Conway; one of my dear friends, Thresea Smith; and finally, *my son*, Caleb Perez. He was like the breathing Nazi! They had me hooked up to some machine that would beep rather loudly and annoyingly if I wasn't breathing properly, and someone would yell at me, "*Breathe!*" And I thought every single time, *I am breathing, or I'd be dead!*

Caleb took this very seriously. He was sitting to the right of me, holding my hand. The machine was right in front of him. So just as soon as it would go off, he would squeeze my hand and tell me to breathe.

This was all going on. I was not receiving any pain medicine because that can affect your breathing. I was *so* tired. I just wanted to sleep. I could barely open my eyes. At one point, I opened my eyes just a little. I could see the foot of my bed only. I couldn't move my head. I just didn't have the energy. All I could do was lie there and move my eyes a little. I was inspecting what I *could* see. I saw the foot of my bed mostly! I closed my eyes for a minute and opened them back up. There at the foot of my bed stood an *angel. Yes*, an *angel. Now* the next events happened rather quickly, but I remember them in such detail. I first thought, *Why is there an angel in my room? What exactly does this mean?* I closed my eyes and thought maybe I was just seeing things. I opened them back up; *yep*, he was still there. What the heck? He was a very slender man with *massive* wings that had *huge* arches that reached the ceiling, and they came all the way to the floor to a very fine point. Here is the strange thing: he was wearing riding boots—black riding boots that came up to his knees. I could not see his face; it was whited out. I felt like his wings had such power in them, as if he could take up the whole room with them. I just stared at him, and I think he knew I was trying to figure out if he was real or not as just then, he cupped the top of his wings and made them flicker, as if to wave at me.

Suddenly, he started gliding toward me. Mind you, Caleb was still sitting at my right, holding my hand, and the angel was coming right at him. I thought, *Listen, buddy, don't hit my kid with your wings!* I feel like he thought that was funny. He then sat (I guess on Caleb's hand) on the edge of the bed; he took his right wing and made it very small then leaned over me a little bit and tucked it under my left side. I was just lying there, thinking, *OK.* Then he made his left wing *huge*, and at this point, he was over me and wrapped me up in his left wing. I could not see anything. I could still feel Caleb's hand. I believe I squeezed it. I could also feel the presence of the angel on top of me. At this point, I thought, *I have no idea what any of this means. Like, is it my time to go? Or what the heck is he doing? But nonetheless, I am just going to close my eyes and go back to sleep.* That is exactly what I did.

According to my mom, after relaying the story to her and discussing what conversations I overheard and who was in the room, this seems to be about the time that I started breathing on my own.

It took me a few weeks to tell *anyone.* I replayed it over and over in my mind, thinking, *Did I make that up?* I asked many questions of my family, such as, "Did I have any pain medicine that could make me see things?" and, "When did I start breathing on my own?", I can tell you today that what I saw was real. It happened. It happened for a reason. I received that visit, and it has given me such peace. God sent me an angel. *Me!*

For some reason after my recovery, I was determined to get a tattoo. I have no idea why. I *never* wanted one before. I knew what I wanted in my mind—the breast-cancer symbol wrapped in angel wings. But the wings had to be just right. I also wanted the words *faith*, *hope*, and *love* to be in the wings. The words didn't happen. I did, however, get the tattoo as soon as I was released to do so after my chemotherapy. Then suddenly, a year later, I had this idea. My best friend, Cheryl Krug-Laskey, is a calligrapher. I decided to have her write the words for me and have the tattoo artist incorporate them around my existing tattoo. Cheryl and I took a napkin, of all things. She traced the existing tattoo, and then she worked on the words. I now have my best friend's words written on my back. I love it!

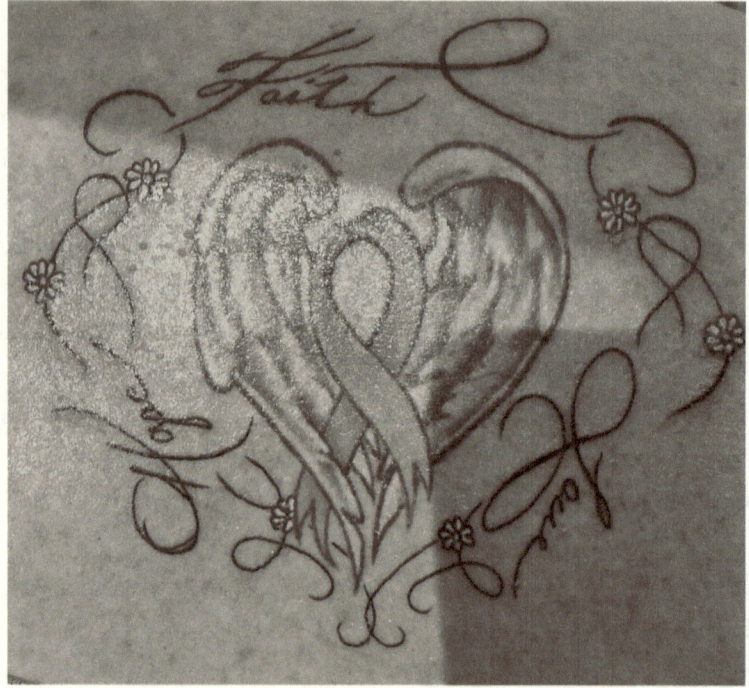

You can see!

Chapter 7

"Caregivers"

This chapter is devoted to the caregivers. I can't tell you how important it is to have someone that can take care of you emotionally and physically.

Caretakers can be your family members, your friends, someone from your social network, or anyone else who helps you through this. Sometimes it can just be someone out of the blue that says something inspirational when you are in a bad place and that can turn you around the other way.

Let me tell you, when I was diagnosed, my doctor and my mom cried. I was not shocked, and I was ready for it. I had already prepared myself for that answer and, quite frankly, would have been shocked if she said it was *not* cancer. So in *my* mind, I just wanted to know what to do next. I was in survival mode. My mother, however, just heard that *her daughter had cancer.* I never really thought of it as something I wasn't going to be able to beat. But as a mother, I understood I also would have been totally frantic if I was in her place!

Then came my telling my seventeen-year-old son, who I just uprooted from his home while I was going through a divorce with his dad, that *now* his *mother* had *cancer.*

He told me that his first thought was *My mom is going to die!* He continued thinking that until we saw the surgeon, at which time he was waiting to hear from her how long I had to live. Of course, that was never discussed because it was treatable.

I believe that we all still have it in the back of our minds. Could it come back? But for the most part, we all live a normal life and have put the cancer behind us.

I don't know what I would have done without my mom and dad taking care of me. The care after the mastectomy was tedious work and taunting. The chemo was scary. But they had to be strong for me although I know they were worried sick about me. I had special care from my cousin Denise. She was kind enough to help take care of me. I have been lucky to have a good support group. Unfortunately, going through a divorce and being unemployed were all difficult things to cope with as well. But when you have cancer, sometimes I think your body just automatically goes into that survival mode.

I would like to acknowledge all caregivers. I applaud you. I *love you* for your patience; your constant giving; your care; and your ability to hold us when we need you, leave us alone when need to be alone, ignore our irritability, cater to our whims, take us to the places we need to go, sit with us patiently at our doctor appointments, listen to us, talk to us, change our bandages, lift us out of bed, take us to the bathroom, lie with us, push us in our wheelchairs, make us laugh, understand when we cry, put all our needs above your own, and tolerate our unexplainable behaviors, but mostly, I *love* you for just being *you*, for putting yourself in the position to be a caregiver. I personally, for myself to my family and for all my friends who helped me along the way, *love* you for helping me make it. I would also like to say for those who are no longer here that I *know* that they thank their caregivers, their families, and their friends. *You* are all special to us, more than you know!

Having said that, I will end with this.

My hope was to inform you of my experience and give you some idea of what happens when you have been diagnosed with breast cancer. I hope that I have helped you in some way. I remain cancer-free for almost three years now. I take a cancer-preventive drug called Femara. I shall continue to take that for two more years. I won't lie; your life will never be the same. Most everyone I know that has had cancer refers to life "BC," *before cancer*, and "AC," *after cancer*. It's not all a bad thing. You are just a different person.

I find that I look at things totally different than I did before. Life is very precious. I don't sweat the little things as much. I pay attention to the things that I love the most. I strive to do what I feel I am meant to do here.

I will also say that sometimes cancer does bring some interesting twists in relationships. If you find that friends or family or spouses are turning away from you, I have learned that some people just don't know how to deal with someone who has cancer. They just can't. So they stay away. Some never come back.

I think that all things happen for a reason. We are put in the places that we are put. We are dealt the cards we are dealt. We receive the gifts we are given, and we struggle to get those gifts sometimes. Sometimes we don't even know when we are receiving a blessing from God until later when it becomes crystal clear. I consider my cancer a blessing in many ways. I know that sounds very strange, but there are so many things that have happened and so many people I have met and been truly blessed by because of it, and I wouldn't have been had I not had cancer.

May God and his angels help you along your journey

www.ingramcontent.com/pod-product-compliance
Lightning Source LLC
Chambersburg PA
CBHW050421290526
45786CB00003B/1360